Outbreak to Pandemic

A Survival Guide

Avoid Infecting or Becoming Infected

A users-guide for everyday people to use in protecting themselves against illness from infectious disease in the community and in making sure they don't cause illness in others.

by

Jared E. Florance, MD, MS, FACPM (emeritus)

1

TABLE OF CONTENTS

Introduction

This book is a self-help guide for you to use in avoiding infectious disease in your community. A self-help for self-preservation.

It is sometimes hard to know what to do and how to feel about reports of an infectious illness in your community. When media reports seem threatening, it is natural to be concerned. Are you and your loved ones truly at risk of serious illness or death? Is it just everyday seasonal influenza, and you are safe because you have had your immunization? Is it "big brother" trying to inflame fear of for political purposes? Is someone trying to sell you something? Is disaster on the horizon? What should you do?

At the time this book is being written, a new coronavirus is being experienced at epidemic levels in multiple countries, and has potential to reach that level in the U.S. You will find answers to many of your "What should I do?" questions as you read on.

You can learn how to answer those questions for yourself. If you use some simple personal infection control habits consistently, the list of illnesses you need to worry about gets smaller. The smaller the list becomes, the easier it is to place a novel situation in perspective. It becomes easier for you to decide whether you need to do anything differently. This book will help you shorten that list and build that perspective. If a new situation could affect you, you will learn how to choose any steps you and your family might want to take to protect yourselves.

Cameo-

400 Kids

It was about 10:00 a.m. when the call came in from a middle school principal. It went something like this:

> "Doc, I have 400 kids puking in the halls. We are closing the school. We think it's the pizza. Can you help?"

After assuring him that we would help, we got to work. We had just begun to marshal our resources when the next call came in, this time from a TV news channel. A camera crew was in route to the school, and they asked for comments.

Can you imagine many things that would be more frightening to a parent than hearing a TV news station talking about a mass outbreak of illness at their child's school? And hearing nothing directly from the authorities other than a statement that "they were looking into it"? We pleaded for time to investigate, and were given until 5 p.m. At that time, the Superintendent of Schools and I met with the reporters and the cameras and gave our report, which fortunately was a calming one.

Over the course of the intervening hours, an immense amount of thought and effort was put into coming up with the right answer. It is a tribute to ALL the members of the school system and the Public Health community that the right answer could be obtained in such a short time. Fortunately, the news was good, given the inauspicious call. Now, more than two decades later, this would more quickly be identified as a probable Norovirus outbreak, much like those reported on cruise ships.

Middle School

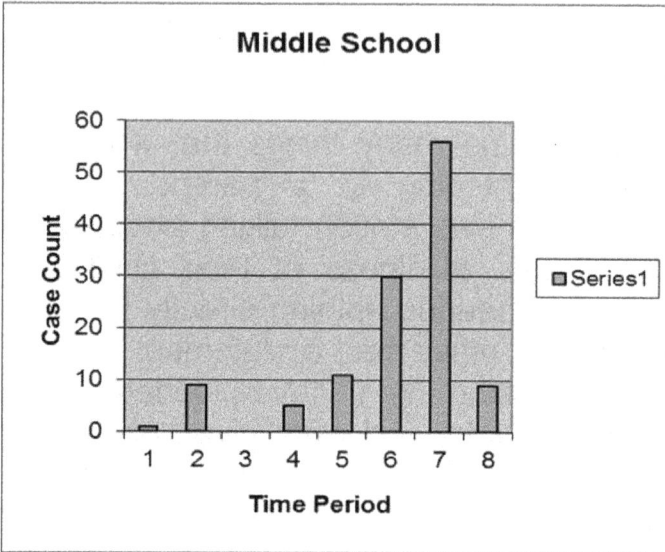

The above graph shows how quickly the new case counts were increasing before new cases suddenly stopped being seen. Each time period was about 12 hours long. A discussion in more detail is in the Appendix.

That was thirty years ago, and Norovirus outbreaks were less common. Now, "tincture of time" has changed how we are affected by these reports. The fear is reduced, if not gone, and such illness is perceived by the community much like a cluster of bad colds.

This huge change in perception is not a bad model for how you will find your own view of illnesses in your community will change as you learn more about them and spend time thinking beforehand on how you will respond if they affect you.

A Day in Your Community

Okay, I admit it isn't **your** community. It is a made-up composite of many communities being used to illustrate some situations you may see in your own.

To give you an idea about how good disease-prevention habits can help you, let us assume for a moment you regularly "cover your cough," and carry a handkerchief (or tissues) and a small bottle of hand sanitizer. You regularly wipe the handle of your shopping cart at the grocery store with the sanitizing wipes most groceries provide. If you use a public restroom, you wash your hands before leaving, and use the towel you dry your hands with to open the door before placing it in the trash can now usually available within reach of the door. You may have a mask tucked in with your other items but have never used it.

Let's start out by having breakfast. Did you know that cases of Hepatitis A, E. Coli (OH157), cryptosporidium and other pathogens have been caused by contaminated strawberries, raspberries, melons, lettuce and other foods you may be putting in front of your family? It is not common, but it does happen. How should you protect yourself? Or should you even worry about it? After all, you must eat, and the cases are few even if they are becoming more frequent. It depends on how well health officials in your community are resourced to manage food safety and investigate any cases of related illness. More on that issue later.

After breakfast, let's take a walk to the park so your toddler can enjoy some fresh air. (Even grandparents, siblings, aunts and uncles get to do this from time to time.) Your toddler notices another child of the same age, and they play. The other child is coughing and sneezing and wiping his or her nose on a sleeve. Your child is the next to play on the same piece of equipment. Could your child have just been exposed to whatever is bothering the other child by the coughing or sneezing, or perhaps by contamination of the hand grips on the equipment? How quickly should you wipe your own child's hands? Will contamination from the equipment be transferred to your child's mouth or eyes by his or her own hand? Maybe you do not have to rush to do something. In most cases, this would just be the usual means by which a child's immunity is built, and some illness is expected with toddlers. Just know whether something especially hazardous is circulating **before** you suddenly find you need to respond to such a situation. It is much more comforting to have done your homework ahead of time. Since you have a handkerchief and your hand sanitizer, you can intervene if you decide it is for the best.

After the park, let's walk to a friend's apartment, and from there take the Metro (subway) to lunch and a movie. When you lock up your house, do you shake the knob to make sure it is locked? Do you know the state of the last hand to grasp that knob? Have you just contaminated the hand you will now use to rub your eye? Is this a good time to sanitize your hands with your hand sanitizer? The same question holds at your friend's apartment. Is there an outer door with a handle you must actuate? Is it a clean handle? Have you now added to its contaminated state with what was on your own doorknob? Again, germs are all around us all the time. Most of the time they are normal community pathogens of no consequence. Some may make you mildly ill. In most cases, frequent hand washing throughout the day is the best way to minimize how often you become ill yourself. When there are several significant illnesses around, such as during flu season, frequent hand washing augmented by use of hand sanitizer may make a big difference.

You walk down the hallway to your friend's apartment, and someone is standing in front of another door, coughing with a wet congested sounding cough. Drug resistant Tuberculosis is making a comeback in the U.S. Is it in your community? Are there an unusual number of cases of pneumonia being seen? Does the air in the hallway seem fresh? Can you tell if the hallway is well ventilated? Some infectious particles can hang in the air for hours. Know what is around, and you will feel in control of the situation. Your handkerchief, pressed over your nose and mouth, can be used as a "field expedient" mask if you decide on extra caution.

Similar questions about exposure to pathogens in the air arise on the subway. The further you travel from your own community, the less sure you may feel about your risks. If it is a particularly bad influenza season, and you have not had this year's flu shot, you might want to consider having a simple mask in your pocket you can put on when the person next to you starts to cough or sneeze. If necessary, your handkerchief could again come into use if a lot of coughing and sneezing is around you.

At the restaurant you use the public restroom before you sit down for your meal. The same questions apply. Did you have to touch the knob with bare hands after you washed them? Was a trash can near the door, so you could use the paper towel you dried your hands with to turn the knob then dispose of the towel? Was there even a towel, or were you only offered a blow dryer? Did you use your hand sanitizer to cover any deficiencies? Did you sanitize your hands after handling the menu, or did you just take your chances on what the last few customers using the menu before you might have left on it? Does it look like restaurant staff are observing good hygiene practices? Do any of them seem ill? If there is a salad bar, are other customers observing good practices when getting their salads? Such things as overall and restroom cleanliness, wellness of staff, and food temperatures and doneness when you are served are among the things you might consider if the restaurant is or might become a regular place for you to dine.

After lunch you head to the theater. It is full, and the first seats you choose are in front of someone that is sneezing or coughing. As you sit, you can feel a damp blast hit the back of your neck. Do you know what is going around? Did you just breathe infectious particles? Did you notice the coughing and put your mask on, or did you ask the attendant for a different seat before sitting down? How you handle the situation may determine whether you become ill or not.

After the movie, you head home, dropping your friend off the on the way. As you get ready to open your door, you wave to your neighbor, who is just helping her elderly mother out of her car and into her house. She comes over later and tells you her mother had been in the hospital with an infection that nearly killed her. She was infected with something sounding like 'Mersa.' You recognize the term from your previous reading as MRSA, Methicillin Resistant Staphylococcus Aureus. You have read that it is a very hard to eliminate infection now being seen in the community. Where a few years ago it was only seen in a few unlucky hospitals, it has become more common. You probe a little and are told that your neighbor was not given any information on the subject. You decide to do some more reading and discuss what this means for you with your own physician or the health department since your children play at her house.

Later, relaxing with your family you reflect about the day and wonder how many opportunities to become infected you avoided because you had good infection-avoiding habits and were aware of what was in the community. You conclude that the habits you have work for you and decide not to change anything. Would you feel the same way if you did not yet have some of those habits?

Some degree of illness is expected in most families, and for growing children it is a time they need to be building immunity. All to often, children are too quickly placed on an antibiotic. This both blunts their bodies effort to build immunity and helps promote antibiotic resistance. As family members age or develop chronic illnesses, even common colds can become dangerous. Knowing the health situation of those in your family will help you avoid putting them in situations where they may become ill. It is when you might become exposed to potential illness in activities outside the home, or when illnesses are brought into your home that you must think more carefully about avoiding infection. In the following chapters, some of the ways you can be exposed will be explored, as will simple habits that might help you avoid exposure. Various ongoing programs in the community to help keep you safe will be discussed. Most questions will have already been considered by the medical and public health communities, but their recommendations may not have made it to you.

The correct answers to a question in Public Health may not fully relieve community concerns. Take the Anthrax letters in the National Capital Region. There were five cases of pulmonary Anthrax, with two fatalities, and 3 million cases of 'terror'. After all, it was a terror attack, and in that sense was quite effective. Such attacks are designed to make people fearful, and it succeeded. Many people took prophylactic antimicrobials because they could not be convinced that they were unexposed. The health care system was strained by the workload imposed by the worried but unexposed. The episode did show America something about its secret weapon against epidemics of infectious disease and bioterrorism - the private medical community. This will be explored later in the Cameo on Anthrax in the Washington Area.

When SARS (Severe Acute Respiratory Syndrome) appeared, it got ahead of control efforts for a while in Canada but was eventually stopped. Good Public Health practice and the cooperation of hospital staffs and of a lot of people in the communities turned the tide. When a case of SARS occurred in a neighboring county to ours, it was stopped with that one case. That quickly, word on how to deal with SARS had been spread. People knew what to do to keep from getting it and had the self-discipline to protect themselves and others. Being aware of what may be circulating in your community helps keep you safe.

Many of the lessons we will be discussing were derived from the experience of episodes like those. Communicable disease takes its name from how it spreads. It is communicated from one person to another by one or more of a few well understood mechanisms. We all can have what we need to protect ourselves, our families and our friends. At most we need to adjust our habits to be more reliable in doing what we already know we should be doing. The hardest part may be to know how much to do, and when, so that we don't become lax at the wrong time because we were too vigilant when there was no need.

Why Should We Think About This NOW?

In addition to what is currently spreading worldwide, there are now frequent reports of common bacteria that have become resistant to antibiotics typically used for them. Foodborne outbreaks of disease occur more frequently, as are recalls of foods from respected large manufacturers. We seem to be in a period where terrorism is on the rise, but it is mostly knives, guns and bombs (and now cars and trucks) that are being seen. Rarely is there talk of infectious agent use by terrorists. The bioterrorism and Smallpox scares of the 1990's and early 2000's have become history. We survived Anthrax, SARS, and Pandemic Influenza (in the form of the Swine Flu in 2009). Ebola breaks out but is more contained, and a new vaccine is being used to protect the involved communities. Smallpox was never released, but outbreaks of monkeypox are ongoing in Africa. These factors complicate the picture as we respond to coronavirus, but do not pose overwhelming barriers to a response. It may be stopped before it gets to your community but discussing it and doing some planning now

21

will help you with the next one to arise as well.

The biggest risk for becoming seriously infected still seems currently to be by one of the agents normally found in your community whose sensitivity to antibiotics, virulence, infectivity or response to immunization is evolving. Influenza is still likely to cause more fatalities than coronavirus in the U.S. this year. Organisms resistant to treatment with antibiotics are more common. Common skin caused by these resistant organisms are more difficult to treat. New mosquito-borne viruses like Zika are causing new patterns of illness. Tick-borne diseases like Lyme disease are more common. As the population becomes more densely packed, spread of some infections from person to person is becoming more common. It is possible that the most important infection for you to avoid is the one you might pick up from the handlebar of the grocery cart at your store, or the knob on a public restroom door.

Cameo-

"It's just infectious disease"

Not long after the Tokyo subway nerve agent attack, a meeting was convened in the Washington, D. C., area to educate local officials and responders about the risks associated with chemical and biological terrorism. Many of the briefings were themselves terrifying. As planning and educating began in the D. C. area, the message too often seemed to be "we are all going to die." An older physician from the local community came forward after a lecture at a local hospital, a lecture that must have had too much doom and gloom in it. He asked why the big fuss? Bioterrorism was, he said, "just infectious disease." His point was that physicians were experienced with controlling outbreaks of infectious disease, and that they would deal with unexpected diseases as a matter of course. Understanding that fact caused a change in how presentations were structured and was a key moment in separately addressing control of disease from control of terror in our thinking and planning. In retrospect, we realized that along the way we had moved from an INTELLECTUAL understanding of the realities involved to an EMOTIONAL ACCEPTANCE that the planned responses would work. It turned out that older physician was right. As shown by the medical and public health response to Anthrax and SARS, it *was* "just infectious disease."

Terror was a state of mind we could learn to manage, and we did. Learning to be aware, and even to be fearful without terror takes time. How many families decided to change their plans for a pregnancy when the media circulated pictures of the first babies with Zika virus infections? Evaluating the ramifications for you of new disease patterns that might affect your community is best done in the clear light of day, before you are affected directly. Clarity in the day will lessen your chance of succumbing to terror in the night. If you have or develop good habits, you have less chance of waking in the night worrying about whether you forgot to wash your hands or were exposed accidentally to a harmful organism.

We cannot predict when something new will arise, when something old will return in a more dangerous form or when something will be released intentionally. We do know at the agency level that it is PARTICIPATION IN THE PLANNING PROCESS, not just the plan, which makes a successful response possible. At home this planning process can be much simpler than for a community. In a medical event at home, people sometimes pull out a thick medical guide and search for an answer before seeking professional advice. When you have thought through what you would do in common situations, the book is more likely to stay on the shelf. When the unexpected occurs in a community, it is too late for the Emergency Manager to pull out the 3-inch-thick binder containing the Emergency Response Plan that someone else wrote and finally start reading it. Those who were deeply involved in the planning effort already have a sense of what must be done. They are the ones most likely to get it done right. The biggest lack of planning involvement may be among the millions of families who have been led to expect that government will protect them. Government will not be able to do everything alone or by directive. Do your own planning for yourself and family, and you will be doing it right.

Given the changes in the diseases circulating in various communities, there will likely be discussions in the media of something new and "dangerous." If there is a problem, it must and will be dealt with. You are already thinking about self-preservation from infectious disease since you are reading this book. This book is for those who wish to be part of the solution to any problem that arises, and not be part of the problem. The solution begins with you. Involving family and close associates in thinking through options ahead of time may make all the difference you need. For even simple community acquired infections, avoiding infection works best if everyone has the same good habits.

On a personal level, thinking about the problem ahead of time will give you time to build the intellectual understanding and plans you need. Moving from intellectual understanding to emotional acceptance will occur naturally over time as your subconscious reviews what you have considered and planned. It will test your efforts on non-threatening events you learn about in the news. The validation and confidence you gain from this process may make all the difference you need to keep your sense of perspective and to keep your fear under control. There will be many happenings that at first seem foretell disaster, but which will again turn out to be false alarms. If something really does turn out to be bad, you will have a much better chance of success than those who were less thoughtful.

The Medical Community Can Treat Infectious Disease

Because of extensive planning and preparation, the National Capitol Region was reasonably well prepared for the Anthrax letters in October 2001. As a result, actual sickness and death were minimized. The attack and its aftermath contained many lessons to be learned.

Cameo-

Anthrax in the Washington Area

Shortly after the first Anthrax case in Florida, I received an after-hours call from an Emergency Room physician who had a very sick patient. The physician had been keeping up to date and recognized the potential for this being the area's first Anthrax case. There were enough red flags raised in our discussion that Anthrax had to be ruled out. Treating this case as a potential Anthrax case involved implementing the terrorism response plan, which in turn meant involving the Federal Bureau of Investigation. Only the State

Health Commissioner had the authority to release enough medial information to the FBI to allow them to evaluate the case for any links to a possibly related case in Florida. After obtaining that authorization, a three-way conference call was held between the Emergency Room physician, the FBI operations center and me. The call confirmed the possibility of a link, and that testing should be done. The specimen was quickly collected and transferred to a State Police officer, who transported it at great speed to Richmond, where the State Laboratory staff quickly tested it. In just a few hours it was determined that it was not Anthrax. But the system had been tested and worked! A few days later, when the area's first Anthrax case was admitted to Fairfax Hospital, Anthrax was diagnosed in time to save the patient. Radiology, the laboratory, the Emergency Room, the physicians and the nursing staff all knew what to do and did it efficiently and effectively.

Even more importantly, they shared everything from imaging results to lab procedures widely in the medical community. When a case was unexpectedly seen in Winchester, some miles away, the medical community was prepared. Anthrax was quickly diagnosed, and the patient survived. All three cases in Virginia survived a disease with a known high mortality. As the event progressed, it was the medical community that conducted the daily regional telephone conferences that became a major communications mechanism in the response.

Local, state and federal Public Health agencies' efforts were closely linked to the efforts of the private medical community. Many patient specimens were tested, environmental samples collected and tested, and an epidemiological understanding of the event constructed. Clinics were established to provide prophylactic antimicrobials to those needing them so that Emergency Room resources could be relieved. The Strategic National Stockpile provided antimicrobials and other materials in its first major use. The various agencies and their plans were tested and found to be sufficient to the task.

Can you see why I think the private medical community is our "secret weapon"? As mentioned earlier, SARS was stopped in its tracks when it arrived in the area. The private medical community in the U.S is exceptional and can be expected to always be leading the response to a biological agent making people ill.

Remember the false alarm? Nothing said above should be construed to lessen the importance of what the Public Health community and other public agencies had done to prepare for such an eventuality. Laboratory testing was available because the Centers for Disease Control, the various state and federal laboratories and various research facilities had developed, distributed and practiced testing methodologies targeted to this purpose. A Strategic National Stockpile of pharmaceuticals and other medical supplies had been created and was the source of the prophylactic antibiotics so widely distributed. Law enforcement had plans to investigate any man-made outbreak and to provide any special security needed during a medical response. The Emergency Medical Services community (mostly fire department rescue squads) was prepared to handle highly infectious cases.

A great deal of Continuing Medical Education had been conducted to bring physicians and others in the medical community up to speed before the event. Health Departments were screening cases for unusual events, and physicians were discussing unusual cases with Health Officers.

The message here is that neither the public sector nor the private sector could have done it without the efforts of the other. It took visionaries in government to get preparations underway. Dedicated professionals in the Public Health, law enforcement and emergency response communities implemented those visions as capabilities, operational plans and daily activities, and began the training process in the medical community. The private medical community implemented the needed capabilities in its area, and when the time came the two sectors were partners in the solution. The same process is undertaken every time something new and dangerous to the community is noticed.

As the coronavirus epidemic progresses, and potentially becomes a pandemic, the preparations that have been made by both the public and private sectors have been up to the challenge.

The missing sector in 2001 was the population itself. While efforts had been made to educate the community about these threats, much of the education tended to make people fearful without giving them a means to be part of the solution. Having a prepared population was a high priority goal that had not yet been met. It is not a goal that can be met by government. It can only be met by members of the community taking ownership and acting both as individuals and as members of the community. Following through on what you read here is a good start.

With the spread of antibiotic-resistant organisms in the community, this kind of engagement by everyone in the community is even more necessary. There is no simple process that can be undertaken by government or industry. Prevention is better than cure, and prevention in this case means everyone having good habits that makes the spread of infectious disease less likely. This is where you come in.

When You Hear Hoofbeats Think Horses Not Zebras

There is an old saying in medical school that when you hear hoofbeats in the night, think of horses not zebras. After studying every disease known to mankind, students often internalize what they have learned by trying to diagnose those diseases in their patients. When it comes time to diagnose the illness that corresponds to the signs and symptoms the student sees, the correct diagnosis more often is found when common things in the community are considered first. We have lots of horses in the U.S., but not many zebras.

As you read about all the diseases described later, and start thinking about how to avoid them, remember that most of them will never be seen in your area. Start with the ones you know are around you and be aware of new diseases moving into the community. Just take pictures of the zebras in a zoo.

Typical Community Illnesses in Today's World

Have you ever noticed that elementary school teachers never seem to be sick? Besides often being among those with the healthiest lifestyles, they also tend to build their immunity early in their careers. Even though their students often catch whichever upper respiratory infection is going around, the teacher may have had it in an earlier year and is immune to re-infection.

Endemic diseases, ones that are always in the community, are the "horses" mentioned above. Not all are "friendly. If malaria or tuberculosis is endemic in your area, there are precautions against infection you should take. Even though uncooked eggs are known to be frequently contaminated with salmonella, GI infections are most easily avoided by proper cooking of eggs and raw meat. In this group, consider common endemic diseases and the infection control habits most people already know how to deal with. These include (but won't be discussed here):

Common Upper Respiratory Infections

"Colds," earaches and similar viral Infections

Influenza

Strep Throat

Bronchitis

Pneumonia and Walking Pneumonia

Meningitis and Encephalitis

Sexually Transmitted Diseases

"Food poisoning"

It is probably not surprising that some of these same diseases can cause outbreaks, epidemics and pandemics when they show up in excessive numbers, with more severe disease, or appear in an area where they had not been seen in recent times. In such cases, a community response is often implemented.

Plagues, Pandemics, Epidemics, Outbreaks, and Endemic Disease

In the strictest sense, Plague is an infection caused by Yersinia (also named Pasteurella) pestis. It has a form spread by fleas (Bubonic Plague) and a form spread person to person (Pneumonic Plague). Plague was responsible for the Black Death in the middle ages. In a broader sense, plague has become a term commonly used (or misused) to reference any calamitous spread of disease, locusts, etc. For our purposes here, epidemic is a more useful word to describe disease suddenly appearing on an unexpected scale. Outbreak is often used to a cluster of cases exceeding expectations locally but not reaching epidemic proportions. An outbreak can be just a few cases for a disease that is rarely seen. Epidemic is used to describe more widespread occurrences. The number of cases it takes before epidemiologists start calling an outbreak an epidemic depends upon the circumstances. A pandemic is an epidemic on a global scale. The terms themselves don't speak to severity of disease, just the patterns of disease being seen compared to what was expected. The H1N1 Pandemic of 2009 was simply not as severe as the Spanish Flu Pandemic of 1918. Our county experienced a Measles outbreak that illustrates several concepts that will be discussed later.

Cameo-

Measles

Measles was diagnosed in a student whose measles case was not classical. It appeared to be a symptomatic but not of typical severity, and it was in someone immunized according to the standard of the time. Few young physicians had seen real measles, since it had essentially been eliminated in the U.S. with a good immunization program. An older, well experienced physician was suspicious, and ordered measles serology, which came back positive.

Over the next several weeks, cases of measles began appearing in other schools. Of note was the early appearance of a large cluster of cases in the same middle school that experienced the gastroenteritis outbreak. The outbreak spread from school to school via siblings in different schools, sports teams, teenage dating and other direct contact means. The outbreak was halted by updating the immunization of every student that had been immunized before the age of one year and excluding from school those whose parents refused to have them immunized for whatever reason. Creating herd immunity worked, and promptly holding immunization clinics in each school where a new case was found prevented secondary cases in that school. In all, 110 clinically and lab diagnosed cases were found in 10 schools, and over 5000 MMR (Measles, Mumps and Rubella) immunizations were administered.

Because of this outbreak, and similar experiences in other communities, the CDC immunization recommendations for middle school and pre-college immunizations against measles were instituted. Immunization programs to create herd immunity work!

Factors in Outbreak Severity

To become ill during an outbreak, several things must happen. Someone or something must have the organism and be able to pass it to you. There must be a way it can be spread. You must allow it to pass your own defenses. You must be susceptible. Implicit in this are agent factors that facilitate or hinder spread, interventions that can block spread, and host factors that influence susceptibility. You can do little to control the agent factors. You *can* do things to block it from infecting you, and for many illnesses you can do things to minimize or prevent illness if you become infected. Depending on your role in an outbreak, you may be able to help reduce the number of people who can be the source of the illness for others.

The impact of a disease on the community depends on several things. These include agent attributes, mechanism of spread, severity of disease, and availability of treatment.

Agent Characteristics

The natural history of an infection tells us a lot. Is there is an asymptomatic "carrier" or shedding period, a period when a person is infectious but has not developed any symptoms? It is much harder to stop an outbreak when asymptomatic shedding occurs, because people can pass it to others before it is known that they themselves have an infection. If the agent can cause sub-clinical cases, it will be harder to control through avoidance strategies. A disease that creates such severe illness that it requires extensive hospitalization in intensive care can overwhelm local hospital resources quickly. Is it a viral agent with no treatment and no vaccine, or is there an effective vaccine that can prevent it? Is it a known bacterium sensitive to a cheap antibiotic or is it one resistant to every antibiotic we have? How long is the prodrome, the period from infection to illness? What are the symptoms? What is the expected mortality? What is its immunogenicity? Does it easily cause such an immune response that you never get it again? Can an effective immunization quickly be formulated, or does the agent evolve so quickly you never catch up?

The answers to these questions are used in formulating response plans at all levels. For example, immunization programs have drastically reduced the illness and mortality that used to be caused by measles, tetanus, diphtheria and pertussis, to name a few. Your own plans should take them into account as well. The more severe the impact if you or a member of your inner circle become ill, the more thorough you should be in planning and in implementing those plans.

Agent Propagation

The mechanism by which the agent spreads is important. A few, like Smallpox and Measles, are airborne. They can hang in the air for hours and blow with the wind. There are documented cases where a child with Measles went to a doctor's office with Measles then left after being seen. Three hours later, another child came to the same office and caught Measles from particles still in the air. Others, like Influenza, can be spread easily as aerosols. Droplets sneezed or coughed are suspended in the air but tend to fall more quickly. A six-foot radius is considered to include the average infectious zone.

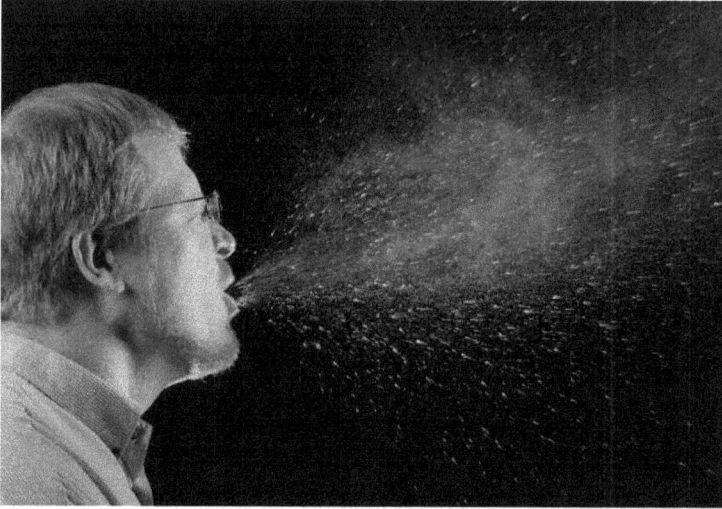

Others, such as E. Coli O157, can be ingested with food or water. West Nile Virus and Zika Virus are injected by feeding mosquitos. Impetigo is caused by Streptococcus or Staphylococcus directly infecting the skin. Both organisms can also cause pneumonia. Streptococci also caused strep throat and Scarlet Fever. Anthrax and plague can also infect through more than one mechanism. How easily an agent can infect a person comes into play when you are in range of a sneeze or cough, ingest it or otherwise come in contact. Does it only take one infectious particle, or can you live with an infected person for a year and still have little chance of becoming infected yourself?

Is the agent easily spread by fomites such as doorknobs and surfaces? Does it convert to a stabile form on the sidewalk that can be kicked up by passers-by and inhaled? Is it acquired by physical contact but infectious only when introduced into an eye, mouth or mucous membrane? Is it able to be suspended in the air by itself or on dust, or must it be in a droplet? How long does it survive outside the body? Old laws against spitting in public were passed because tuberculosis organisms were being spit onto the street, where they were dried by the sun, then kicked up by the feet of passers-by. They could then be inhaled by the next person to pass, and that person could become ill.

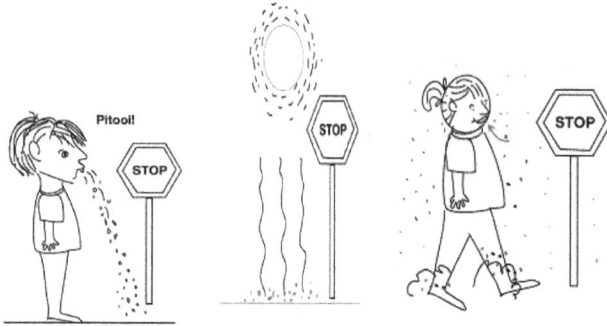

In the 1990's active TB cases were found in children in all three of our school systems. These infected children all infected other children.

Anthrax occurs naturally in many parts of the world but was also used in a bioterrorism event. It does not naturally spread in a way that could cause a Pandemic. In its spore form it is very hardy, and as used in the event easily caused plumes of spores that could be inhaled and cause disease. It spread on clothing, skin and objects, but could be removed by cleaning. By securing and decontaminating affected spaces further spread was prevented.

For new diseases, such as SARS, the public health and medical communities have quickly determined and reported on disease properties and proposed control measures. By learning about how a new disease is spreading, you can pick the practices you need to reduce your chances of becoming ill. If you already have some choices in your "bag of tricks" because you planned to stay uninfected, it will be much easier for you to protect yourself, and the chance you will react to fear lessened.

Host Factors

Different people have different susceptibilities to a disease and will experience a different severity when ill. People with chronic a disease, and the extremely young and extremely old often have more severe cases of Influenza, for example. Up to date immunizations effectively prevent the diseases for which they are designed. Even out of date immunizations can, in some cases, lessen the severity of disease. In our Measles outbreak, the term "symptomatic re-infection" was used to describe cases where the patient's immunity had lessened with the passage of time since immunization, and they became ill as a result. Some of them were infectious but the infections were subclinical in that they did not really appear to be classic Measles. Once the outbreak was confirmed, cancer patients and others with compromised immune systems were warned. Some needed hospitalization and treatment with immune globulin to insure survival. Once an agent is known to be one you could be exposed to, you can estimate your own risk and adjust your *posture* accordingly.

Community Factors

Population characteristics in an area are major determinants of how an outbreak proceeds in the community. A ranch couple in Montana will simply be have less risk of exposure than a large family residing in a forty-story condominium in New York City. The number of people you interact with daily, and the number with which each of them interacts, determine the size of population that should concern you. The higher the level of interaction, the more likely it is for the agent to be able to reach you in an unguarded moment. Even in small communities, people interact. It is your daily activities, such as shopping, going to work or school, meeting with friends and colleagues, and anything else you do with groups that create the opportunity for you to be exposed to the agent involved.

The Impact of Globalism

Several recent food-borne outbreaks were attributed to contaminated foods imported into and distributed in the U.S. Foods that are not cooked, such as berries, are more likely to cause illness if contaminated.

Bioterrorism

Agents distributed in bioterrorism events may not be as easily controlled as Anthrax was in the Washington case. Agents might be picked because they can be distributed mechanically and cause extensive disease where they infect you, but don't efficiently spread disease beyond the original distribution area. Secondary infections can be caused when the organisms are further spread by ill persons, by poor practices by providers, and by the movement of people and equipment through the contaminated area. These features can create the desired terror without endangering the terrorist. Without due care, the response itself can spread the agent. Agents can be carried out on clothes, boots, other objects or with ill cases being evacuated if responders and those fleeing the area are careless.

Threat agents could also be picked because they spread easily person to person. Smallpox was a threat for this reason. As a threat agent, Smallpox would be a two-edged sword. If released, it would have the potential for reaching the terrorists' home country and wreak the same havoc there as at the location of original target.

Changes in the Health Care System

As for-profit medicine continues to cut costs by restricting diagnostic testing, office visits, pharmaceuticals and other tools for diagnosing and treating infections, the ability of the medical and public health communities to respond in a timely manner has been diminished. More on this later, when better context has been established.

Considering the Extreme Situation

There is a wide range of possibilities to consider when a large outbreak of infectious disease occurs. While most outbreaks are controlled easily, a Pandemic would be a challenge. If you can prepare yourself for a Pandemic, you have done something significant. For this reason, much of the ensuing discussion will consider this extreme, which means that any outbreak discussed as if it were part of a severe Pandemic. This doesn't mean that Pandemics are inevitable. Plan for the worst, hope for the best, and expect something in between.

Given that intent, the focus will often be on person to person spread. Pneumonic plague, Spanish Influenza, smallpox and measles are historical examples of droplet and airborne spread diseases communicated person to person. Norovirus, SARS, swine flu and tuberculosis resistant to multiple drugs have all received recent media attention. "Test" any plans you make against the sometimes-intimidating outbreaks seen in various parts of the world. As you follow them in the media you can gain some reinforcement that you are on the right track.

Social distancing measures, management of your environment, personal protective equipment, and personal hygiene measures are major tools at your disposal. Think of the collection of social and personal habits, protective gear, sanitizers, "tightening" of your home and so on that you would use in a severe outbreak as a *posture*. If you think of your own response plans in terms of the *posture* you would adopt for each situation, or for different phases of a Pandemic, you can define as few or as many as you feel will work best for you. Coming up with those *postures*, and your own rules for when to adopt each, is a task you should think about as you read on. Think about the worst-case scenarios as you do this. In each situation, you can always decide nothing extra is needed, but when you have pre-planned options from which to choose, life becomes simpler. In most cases thinking about it will be all you have to do.

A bioterrorism event, being "just infectious disease" would be covered by your plans for a Pandemic event.

Outbreaks involving Person to Person Spread Illnesses

Fortunately, most of the communicable diseases that made children sick in ages gone by have been controlled by immunization programs. Measles, mumps, rubella, pertussis, diphtheria and polio are examples of illness that once caused significant morbidity and mortality in the U.S. but were until recently well controlled by immunization programs.

"Herd immunity," where so many people have antibodies to a disease that the rare cases that occur create no or few secondary cases depends on most people in the "herd" having had the disease or the immunization. This philosophy was the basis for the elimination of smallpox from the world. The total elimination of a disease is difficult for several reasons. Diseases thought eliminated can reappear if immunity in the herd wanes, such as when children born into the "herd" never get antibodies because there is no circulating agent to cause the illness and they never receive the immunization. An infectious visitor to the community can cause an outbreak.

Even those immunized can have "waning immunity" if there is no circulating agent to challenge the immune system and cause it to make new antibody. Waning immunity was an underlying feature of the Measles outbreak referenced in this book. Such outbreaks resulted in additional doses of Measles vaccine being required in middle school and prior to college. The "antivaxxer" movement has also resulted in a reduction in "herd immunity," facilitating the occurrence of outbreaks. Agent evolution or mutation can also be a reason for immunizations to become less effective. In such cases, an updated vaccine is required.

A few of these re-appearing diseases that have caused outbreaks are:

Measles

Measles outbreaks are now occurring with a disquieting frequency. A disease that had been essentially eliminated in the U.S. is again causing significant disease and unfortunate mortality, principally because people are forgetting or had never learned how serious this disease can be and listen too readily to the "anti-vaxxer" propaganda.

A 2019-2020 outbreak of Measles in Samoa had over 5700 cases, with 83 deaths out of a population of 200, 874.

In 2019, Washington State had two outbreaks spanning January to August. Eighty-six cases were identified.

In all, there were over 1000 cases in the U.S. in 2019. Twenty-three States were involved, with New York having the most at almost 700.

Given that at one time Measles was nearly non-existent in the U.S., the combined effects of under immunization, immigration, and tourism on disease increase can be seen.

Tuberculosis

A few decades ago, TB testing was de-emphasized in the U.S. on the belief that it was adequately controlled in the U.S. and that newly imported cases could easily be identified and treated. It was felt that the funds supporting the control program could be reprogrammed to other uses. Relaxed immigration policies have allowed more infectious persons to take up residence in the U.S., and the increasing prevalence of multi-drug-resistant TB in other parts of the world to change the calculus of control.

My Health District experienced clusters in children in all three school districts plus the Juvenile Detention Center. A few cases were resistant to most treatment options and required daily supervised therapy. In at least one case, daily injection was required. Not all patients were compliant with recommendations for controlling spread to others. Legal action was required to prevent further spread in at least one case.

Because of one particular case, a workplace requested TB testing of selected co-workers. Close daily contacts were tested, but when a high infection rate was noted, over 1000 employees were eventually tested.

Pertussis

Pertussis, or whooping cough, can kill infants. In 2012, there were over 48,000 cases in the U.S. The number of cases waxes and wanes.

An acellular vaccine was created to reduce complications. Increases in case number appear to be a multifactorial. There is some waning of efficacy. One study showed the vaccine was only 60% effective. There is some concern that waning immunity in adults and older children could be a factor.

Cases in older persons do not have as much risks as in infants, but infectious adults can still infect infants in close contact. Control programs are more likely to be focused on prophylaxis for contacts with infants in their circle, rather than broad contact programs.

Outbreaks appear to stay within defined populations and given the high level of immunization everywhere else, Pandemic potential does not appear to exist.

Norovirus

Norovirus is often associated with cruise ships. Once thought to be predominately transmitted by the fecal-oral route via contaminated surfaces, etc., it is now known to also be transmitted directly person to person. In two of the outbreaks in our county thought to be Norovirus, there was an apparent spread as an airborne, not just droplet, mechanism. The middle school outbreak described in an earlier Cameo was probably a Norovirus. The fact that our Measles outbreak began in the same school, with a similar "explosion" of cases supports the airborne spread hypothesis.

Fortunately, the Norovirus seen our county was mild illness and burned through susceptible populations quickly, and self-extinguished as a result. Epidemic or Pandemic scale requiring a massive intervention is not likely.

Hepatitis -A

Hepatitis-A has been involved in a long running multi-state outbreak since 2017. CDC lists several risk factors:

People who use drugs (injection or non-injection).

People experiencing unstable housing or homelessness.

Men who have sex with men (MSM).

People who are currently or were recently incarcerated.

People with chronic liver disease, including cirrhosis, hepatitis B, or hepatitis C.

This extended outbreak has involved 32 states and over 30,000 cases.

Hepatitis-A has also been associated with day-care center clusters, in food-borne outbreaks involving berries, and in restaurant associated outbreaks.

Despite the size and persistence of the outbreaks in some at-risk populations, involvement of most groups appears unlikely. Pandemic potential does not exist.

Person-to-Person Summary

In summary, these endemic diseases will continue to cause outbreaks, but are unlikely to be involve in Epidemic or Pandemic scale clusters. Immunization status is important in any group at risk. The Anti-vaxxer movement is causing significant morbidity and some mortality by discouraging proper immunization.

Outbreaks Involving Spread Via Environmental Factors

With globalization, many of our assumptions about our personal environments have become invalid. Most of the risks you now incur can be lessened with thoughtful adjustments to your habits and environment.

Avian influenza and swine influenza have both been in the news as potential Pandemic viruses. A swine flu was the virus in the 2009 Pandemic, but fortunately was not of the severity feared. The potential for severe Pandemic viruses to evolve from these lines is troubling. Any virus that can be spread worldwide by migrating birds, for instance, should be watched closely for its potential to jump to humans in a form that is contagious. Be aware of any such viruses being monitored for new patterns of spread. Not all "animal" risk is from infectious disease.

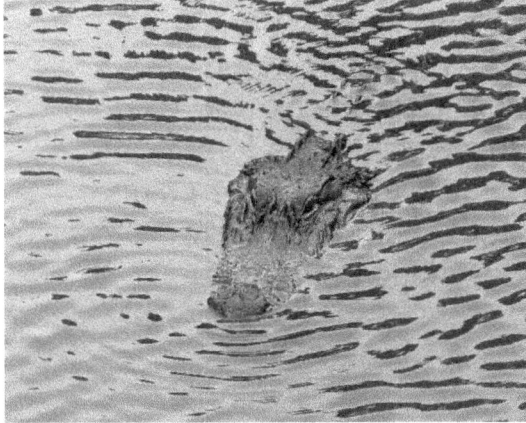

Food

In 1996, there were outbreaks of Cyclospora caused by contaminated raspberries from Central America. In 1997, strawberries contaminated with Hepatitis A found their way into a school lunch program. In a few short years, imports of food products from Central America had grown significantly. The problem was eventually attributed to the hygienic practices of field hands in the involved countries, particularly when illness was present in those workers. People in the U.S.

were so accustomed to safe and clean food that many were caught unaware and became ill. Remember Mad Cow Disease? As farming and animal husbandry practices change there are opportunities for things to go awry. Fortunately, these outbreaks tend to be point-source, sometimes from multiple points, but not propagated outbreaks like the measles outbreak described earlier.

Cameo-

E. coli O157, hamburgers and alfalfa sprouts

Pathogenic E. coli came to national attention when a number of people became ill eating under-cooked hamburgers. The ground beef involved had been contaminated somewhere in the chain between live animal the restaurant where it was served. For this and other reasons, a process for fingerprinting enteric pathogens was developed to use in linking clusters of illness, particularly for foods used widely but sparsely. The first graph shows the cases from the 1993 outbreak based on when they occurred, and the progress of the outbreak over time.

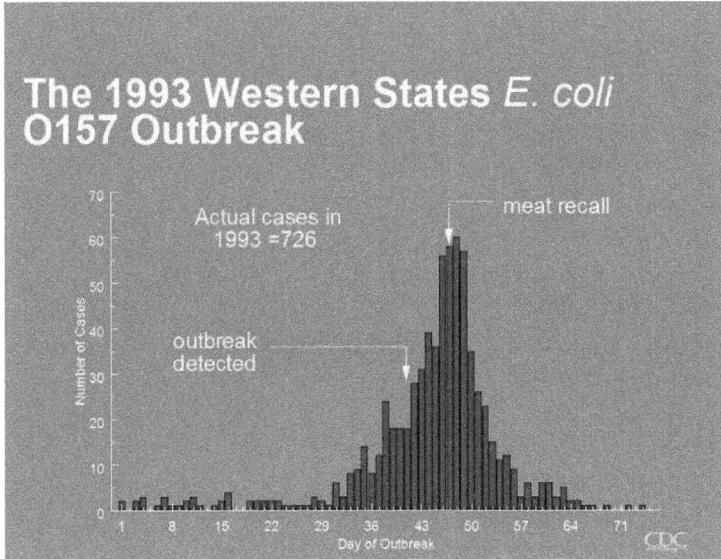

The 1993 Western States *E. coli* O157 Outbreak

The second graph shows how much more quickly the outbreak would have been controlled had it occurred once fingerprinting was in place.

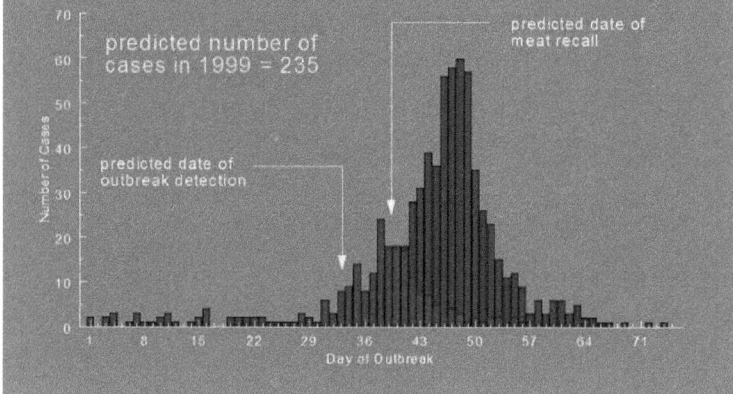

Predicted curve had the outbreak occurred in 1999...

predicted number of cases in 1999 = 235

predicted date of meat recall

predicted date of outbreak detection

Number of Cases

Day of Outbreak

Ever since then hamburger has been the culprit of choice in many persons minds when E. coli caused an outbreak. It turned out that the next outbreak in Virginia was instead associated with Alfalfa Sprouts. It is now known that outbreaks are caused by fruits and vegetables more often than by meat. The illnesses, however, are usually less severe.

Our food supply chain leads from farm to table. The longer that chain, the more opportunities occur for contamination. Restaurants are regulated to prevent illness, but sometimes the regulations have exemptions that allow outbreaks to occur. Our jurisdiction had the misfortune to be the home of a large outbreak where 86 of 115 attendees became ill from the same cause. Food was improperly prepared and stored for a St. Patrick's Day dinner. Those preparing the dinner were exempt from the restaurant regulations.

Hepatitis A cases in food service workers are seen occasionally. Food service workers sometimes work when they are ill, even though restaurant regulations forbid them from doing so. Sometimes they are told to work, and sometimes they choose to work to protect paychecks and even jobs.

The one confirmed food bioterrorism event in this country occurred in Oregon, when members of a sect caused Salmonella to be sprayed on a salad bar at a restaurant. This was a deliberate attempt to make residents ill so that an election could be swayed in favor of the sect. The scale of this type of event is limited by the size of the groups that could be affected before the event was detected and halted. A great deal of government planning has gone into assuring protection from such actions.

The lesson here is that any uncooked or under-cooked food can cause illness, and that outbreaks can be caused when the contamination occurs in the food supply chain, when food is purposefully contaminated or when food is prepared, stored and provided by a source not having proper training or equipment. These outbreaks are generally limited in spread, and while a problem for those who become ill, are not of such scope that they are likely to cause a Pandemic. Person to person spread is not a common feature of foodborne outbreaks.

The use of unpasteurized milk, and products made with unpasteurized milk is increasing. Each year, outbreaks of illness occur when these products are distributed containing infectious agents. Your best protection is to avoid them, and the risk of becoming ill is one you will have to consider if you choose to consume them.

Your protection here is principally awareness and due care. If something you have bought is subject to recall, cooperate with recall instructions. If a press release is held telling you a restaurant had an ill worker and immune globulin is advised for diners, get it if you were one of them. Wash your fruits and vegetables before eating. Keep your cold foods cold, hot food hot, and store and consume or dispose of leftovers as recommended for the type of food involved.

Water

John Snow is considered by many to be the father of epidemiology. He halted a cholera outbreak in London in 1854 when by analyzing cases by residence and place of work was able to identify the Broad Street Pump as the culprit. The Broad Street Pump drew water that flowed to it from the Thames River, water that was being contaminated by human waste being discharged into the Thames upstream from the well. His removal of the well handle ended the outbreak. Flooding from Hurricane Katrina contaminated water supplies in the area. Typhoid and other infectious disease risk had to be considered.

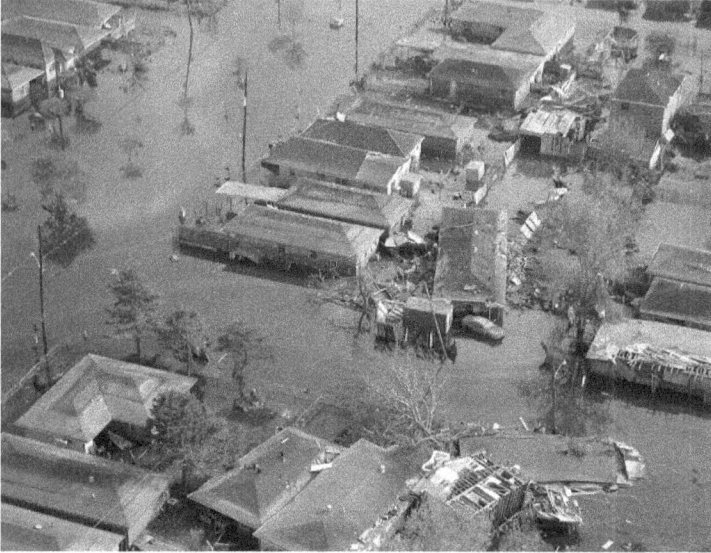

In 1993, over 400,000 persons in Milwaukee, WI, became ill when the public water supply was contaminated with cryptosporidium. The contamination was thought to be naturally occurring in runoff from farms, and not due to any human intent. The water system failed to filter out the organism, which was not killed by the treatment process. This event resulted in a great deal of attention being placed on water supply protection during counter-terrorism planning. Because such events are necessarily limited in spread, and because the matter is so thoroughly addressed by regulatory agencies, your risk from public water supplies is almost nil.

Insects, birds, bats and animals

Most people who live in climes that support mosquito populations are aware of how West Nile Virus came to the U. S. and spread over much of the southeast. Carried by birds, and spread to people by mosquitos, WNV has become endemic. It can cause a severe encephalitis. Because of its potential for outbreaks, extensive efforts have been made to manage mosquito populations and reduce human exposure. There were significant mosquito control efforts undertaken after Hurricane Katrina for this reason.

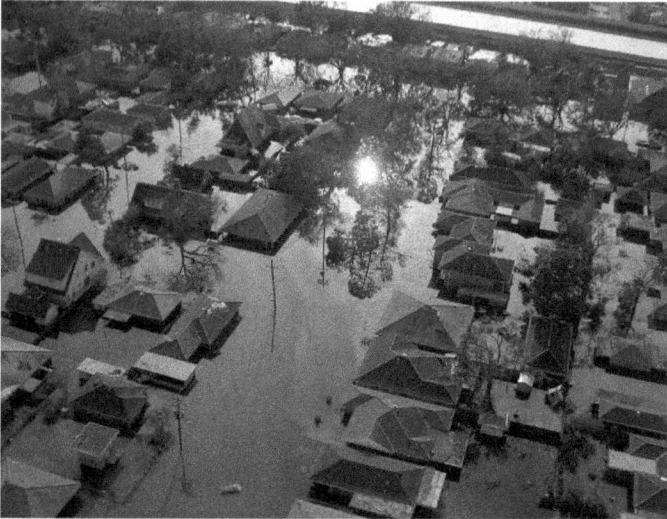

WNV is presented here to illustrate the potential for new agents to naturally become endemic when introduced into the U.S., but also to point out the care that the responsible agencies take in trying to minimize illness from diseases like this. Your thoughts should consider any *endemic* diseases in your area that justify being considered in your posture.

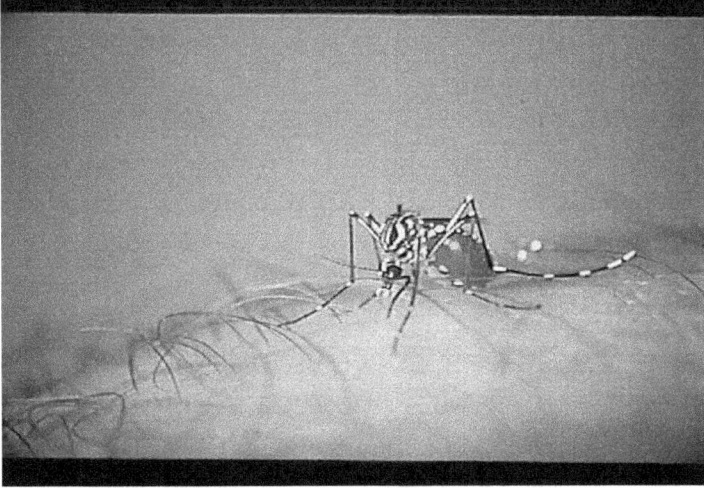

There are enough mosquito-borne, tick-borne and flea-borne diseases in the U.S. that you should know what is present locally, and what you should do should an outbreak occur. Other diseases, such as Rabies spread by bats and raccoons, have become local issues in several states. Local jurisdictions have control and protection programs in place where warranted. Information about what you should look out for and how you should prepare are available from them.

Your best protection when there are serious endemic mosquito-borne diseases in your area comes from following the recommendations for your area as published by health authorities. Keep your house mosquito free with screens. Follow recommendations for preventing breeding sites on your property. During times of day when mosquitos in your area bite, wear proper clothing and use the recommended insect repellent when going outside.

For tick borne diseases, wear long sleeve clothing tight at the wrists and ankles, and do a tick check of your person after venturing out into the woods or fields in your locale. If you find a tick that has been in place for more than a day, contact your health care provider or the Health Department for guidance.

Bats are a special case. Bats are important as insect eaters, and some people put up boxes for them to nest in. Most of the human cases of rabies in the U.S. over the past few decades have been due to a bat rabies variant. A known bite by a bat, or a bat found in a bedroom when waking up, or where a child was unattended or where a disabled person was staying are all grounds for testing the bat for rabies. If it is not available for testing, or if the test is positive, rabies prophylaxis is recommended. Bat-proof your home and be aware of potential bites.

Hantavirus causes a severe pulmonary illness. It is mostly seen in the southwestern U.S. Cases sometimes are seen after people sleep in shelters where mice have left droppings. In an endemic area, any camp, home or workplace can be a place of exposure if mice are present. Find out if hantavirus is a problem in areas where you might have exposures to mouse droppings, and if so, follow local Public Health recommendations to prevent exposures. If you live in an area where hantavirus is endemic, rodent control around your home is your first line of defense. Plug entrances, trap them, and keep your house clean so they aren't attracted.

Birds and animals as hosts for agents affecting humans

Animal and bird reservoirs for agents that have human Pandemic potential are watched closely. In 2003, there was a multistate outbreak of monkey pox in the U.S. when an imported animal infected prairie dogs destined to be pets. No person to person spread was documented. All transmission appeared to have occurred by direct contact with the infected prairie dogs, or the places they were kept.

H1N1 swine flu was the 2009 Pandemic agent. A vaccine was produced, and immunizations given worldwide. In the U.S., small outbreaks of swine flu variants occurred in 2009 centered around petting zoos at fairs. Person to person spread was believed to have occurred, but significant spread did not occur. Animal exhibits were the source of these outbreaks. Swine flu will continue to be monitored closely, and you should maintain an awareness of its status.

H5N1 avian influenza has been considered a prime Pandemic candidate since 2003. With a significant mortality rate, and persistent reservoirs in bird populations in some parts of the world, it lacks only enhanced human to human spread to become a Pandemic agent. Since this is an influenza virus, you would protect yourself using the tools described in this book. Candidate vaccines are available. Every case worldwide is evaluated for the possibility of human to human spread.

Migratory routes are monitored for infected birds carrying the virus. It is expected that should the genetic changes needed for enhanced human spread occur, rapid identification of that fact will allow a timely response. Be aware of any formal announcements that this has taken place.

Potential for non-Pandemic exposure to agents increases when you visit areas where contact with infected birds and animals is possible.

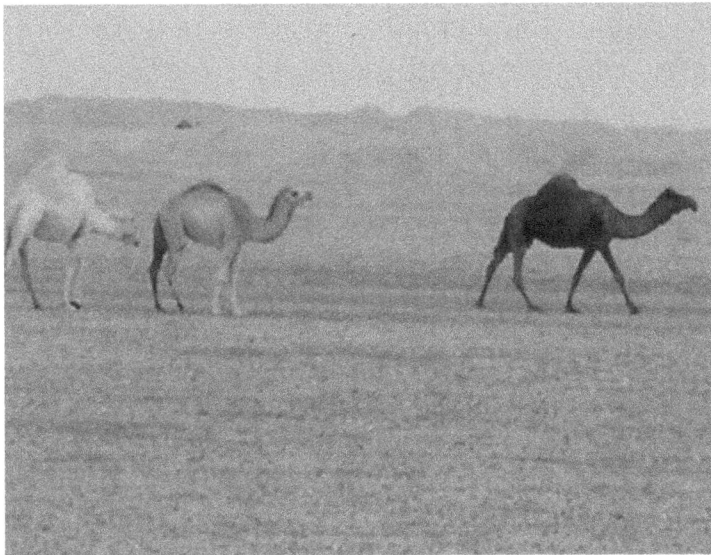

Mid-East Respiratory Syndrome is caused by a coronavirus that appears to be a mutation of a camel virus. It has caused outbreaks in humans, with limited person to person spread. It has been a disease of concern for those planning a pilgrimage to the Mideast, but only a few clusters outside the Mideast have been seen.

Avoid contact with wild birds and animals, particularly if visiting locales where the viruses are endemic. Do not keep wild or exotic animals as pets and avoid places that have them. If you visit animal exhibits, wash your hands carefully after contact with any animals. Ensure any children in your care do the same. Practice good mosquito exposure avoidance if you are in an area with endemic mosquito transmitted agents like West Nile Virus. Immediately adopt all precautions recommended to protect you from exposure to *any* agent of concern present where you live or visit. The CDC make recommendations on their web pages for avoiding exposures to these agents in general, and by country for travelers to other countries.

Soil and Solid Objects

Histoplasmosis can be inhaled from the soil in areas under roosts that have been in one place for too many years. This was found to be the case when a wooded area that had housed a roost for a number of years was cleared for a park. A group camped in the park, and several campers developed pulmonary histoplasmosis.

Coccidioidomycosis is a human fungal infection whose spores can be inhaled with the dust in some areas. It is often called Valley Fever. It is sometimes seen in construction projects in affected areas, particularly in parts of California.

Other diseases caused by mold are experienced in caves, damp buildings, tombs and the like. Care should be exercised to ensure your living space is free from mold, particularly where spores can be circulated by your activities.

There are many things that cause disease in humans, but few of them have pandemic potential.

A Few Public Health Concepts

Prevention

"An ounce of prevention is worth a pound of cure"-Ben Franklin

Public Health is part of the specialty of Preventive Medicine. Prevention is usually referred to in terms of primary, secondary and tertiary prevention. The goal is always to attain primary prevention where possible. For this book, only prevention of infectious disease will be considered.

Primary prevention is where you try to avoid having someone become ill in the first place. Preventing infection is primary prevention. Personal Protective Equipment (PPE) and immunizations are both tools used in primary prevention. If the agent cannot establish a foothold, it cannot make you ill.

Secondary prevention is where you try to avoid some of the seriousness of the event. Taking an antimicrobial to eliminate the infection before it becomes serious is secondary prevention.

Tertiary prevention is trying to heal the person, and to prevent further deterioration. Improving the overall health of someone with extremely drug resistant Tuberculosis so that they can continue to function is tertiary prevention.

Infectious disease

There are several terms that describe aspects of infectious disease that are often used synonymously, when they are different. Communicable disease, for instance, describes a disease that can move from one person to another, but does not specify mechanism. Contagious disease implies direct contact or spread in the air.

A person may be exposed to disease without becoming infected. If the organism establishes a foothold, infection has occurred. A carrier may have an infection that does not turn into disease, but which may be contagious. A person who is ill or recovering but is still infectious is also considered to be in a carrier state. Once an infection affects the individual directly, it has caused disease. The presence of symptoms usually marks this stage. Sub-clinical cases are those where disease is present without the expected symptoms. The person may be infectious before, during, and/or after symptoms are seen, depending upon the organism's characteristics and the natural history of its disease in humans.

Epidemiology

Epidemiology is the study of diseases on populations. An epidemiologist tries to determine all the relevant factors associated with the spread of a disease, and to determine how its spread can be interrupted.

The three graphs that follow illustrate how point-source, propagated and continuous-source outbreaks can be identified by the relationship of the cases to place, time and other cases. How the cases occur is only one of the factors epidemiologists must consider.

How these graphs change over time in response to the disease control interventions used measures the effectiveness of those interventions,

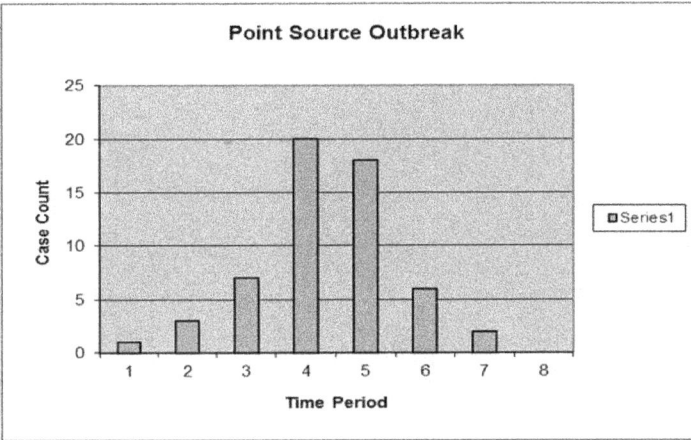

Point Source Outbreak

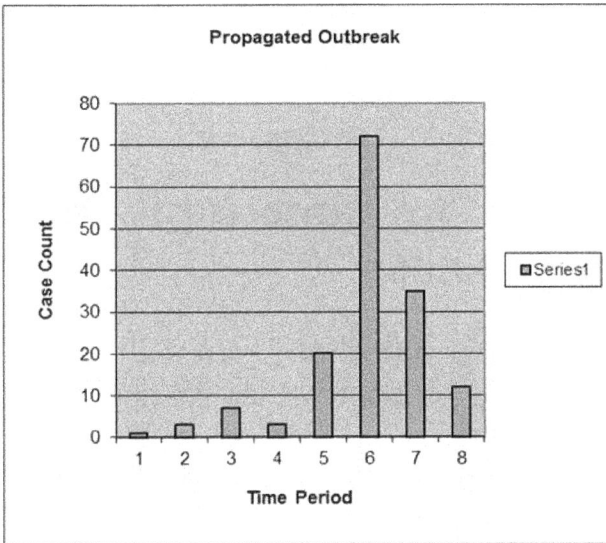

Propagated Outbreak

81

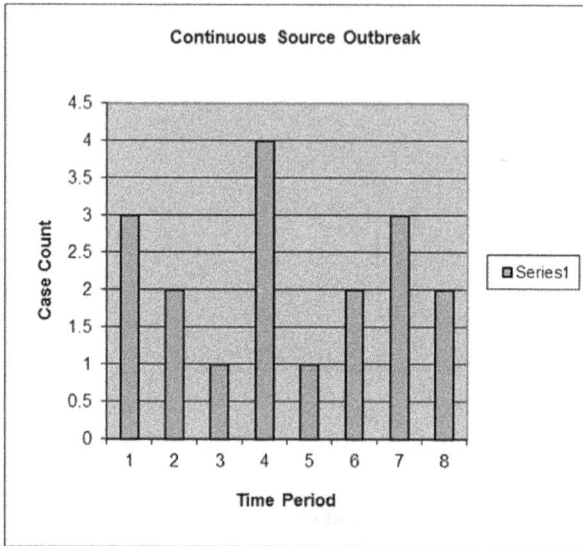

Continuous Source Outbreak

Programs to Interrupt the Spread of Illness

Both non-pharmaceutical and pharmaceutical approaches are important in limiting and ending outbreaks. Social distancing, sequestration quarantine and isolation and isolation all have roles in reducing person to person spread. Post-exposure prophylaxis and immunization programs directly block the person to person spread.

Social Distancing, Sequestration, Quarantine and Isolation

Before we go on to how to protect yourself in your communities, you need to understand the terms used to describe formal actions sometimes taken to limit the spread of infection in and between groups of people. In responding to a Pandemic, every mechanism thought to have merit will be used to buy time while the agent is identified, a vaccine or other approach developed, and immunization and intervention programs implemented.

Social distancing is the term that describes efforts to spread people out, so it is harder for an agent to pass through the community. Meetings may be cancelled. Day care and other group settings for children may be closed. Sporting events may be cancelled, both to protect the athletes and to eliminate the crowds of spectators. The recommended guidelines may change depending upon the agent involved and the demographics of the community.

Sequestration is the formal limiting of access by outside people to an unexposed group having no one ill with the disease in question. During some epidemics in the past, communities have essentially closed their borders to visitors in the hopes of keeping the epidemic at bay. This was rarely effective. Using the concept to design protection strategies for military units, critical infrastructure operators, continuity-of-government designees and other well defined groups where movement and access can be managed has merit. It is critical that the rules for access to a sequestered group be zealously enforced, lest one visitor incubating the disease expose the entire group. It is the difficulty in enforcing these rules that limits the groups for which sequestration will work. Who plans to tell a grandparent or "the boss" that he or she cannot be admitted because of a potential exposure? The term shelter-in-place is used by the Department of Homeland security to describe self-sequestration, which is part of its plan.

Quarantine is the limiting of access to well people by persons believed to be exposed to the disease. Quarantine is enforced until the exposed person becomes ill, or until enough time has elapsed that becoming ill from the exposure is no longer possible. This quarantine period is specific for the disease and will be specified by Public Health officials for the outbreak agent. If a group is in quarantine, and a member of the group becomes ill, the ill person would be isolated, and the quarantine period for the rest of the group restarted. Quarantine is rarely used today. It was, however, used to good effect in stopping SARS in Canada. In an epidemic where a person can become infectious before developing any symptoms or signs of the disease, where treatment is not assured, and where outcomes are poor, quarantine can be an important control tool. Quarantine is being used extensively to control coronavirus.

Isolation is the next step from quarantine. It is used when an ill person can infect others and is usually begun when symptoms are seen. It is the end of infectivity that determines when isolation can be relaxed. Unlike quarantine, where the time period is usually a multiple of the incubation period for the disease, isolation depends both upon the natural history of the disease, and upon the course of the disease in the individual involved. Medical facilities currently impose isolation routinely for selected diseases as part of their infection control plans.

Cameo-

SARS and Isolation and Quarantine

Severe Acute Respiratory Syndrome (SARS) first arrived in Toronto in February 2003. The outbreak eventually included 257 persons in several Greater Toronto Area hospitals. Province wide Public Health measures were imposed, and the outbreak came to an end. The World Health Organization (WHO) lifted a travel advisory it had issued that had recommended limiting travel to Toronto. SARS reappeared in May, about a month after it was thought eliminated. It appears that undiagnosed SARS in hospital patients caused cases in health care workers once the control measures had been relaxed. During the period April to June, 79 more cases were reported, most in health care workers and patients who caught it in the hospital, and the rest in visitors.

Increased measures were implemented, including health care workers being placed on a 10-day work quarantine, instructed to avoid close contact with family and friends, and to wear a mask whenever close contact could not be avoided. Only one of the 79 cases was thought to have resulted from an exposure that occurred after the increased measures were put into effect.

FIGURE 1. Number* of reported cases of severe acute respiratory syndrome, by classification and date of illness onset — Ontario, February 23–June 7, 2003

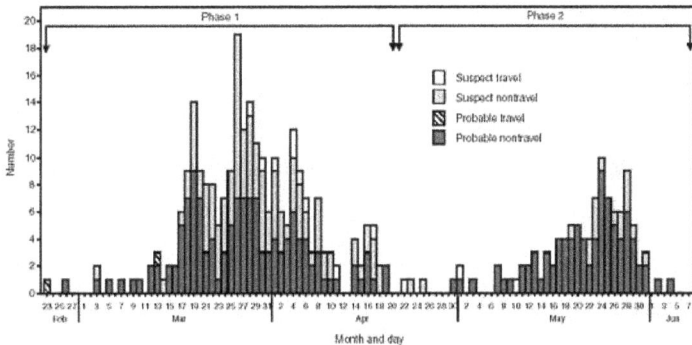

* N = 361.

The chart above, taken from the CDC's **Morbidity and Mortality Weekly Report**, shows the two clusters of cases. Isolation for ill patients, and work quarantine for health care workers were both used in controlling this outbreak.

Public Health law generally provides for the imposition of modified or full quarantine under special circumstances to protect the public. A limited quarantine authority is sometimes in state health regulations to allow unimmunized students to be excluded from school during an outbreak, since exposure can rarely be determined, and there is risk to other students should the unimmunized student become ill. The exclusion of ill food service workers from handling food intended for public consumption is often included in this limited quarantine authority.

Post-exposure Prophylaxis and Immunization

When a case of Meningococcal meningitis occurs, close contacts are often given antibiotic prophylaxis. N. Meningitides, the causative organism, is often carried asymptomatically by people in the general population. Carriage rates as high as one in five persons have been seen in close living situations like military boot camp. In this disease, prophylaxis is intended to protect any infants who might be exposed while their immune systems were still immature. Trying to eliminate the organism widely would not be practical.

In our Measles outbreak, immunizing students whose immunization history suggested they were at risk stopped the outbreak. This outbreak is described in a Cameo later in this book. The Ebola epidemics in Africa have been sharply curtailed with broad use of a quickly developed and tested immunization. Since some strains of Ebola have high mortality rates and are difficult to treat, this vaccine has literally been a lifesaver. With Pandemic Influenza planning, development and distribution of a vaccine has been included as being essential to ending such a Pandemic. Wide protection of the population against seasonal influenza using that season's regular vaccine is an essential part of the strategy since it would speed diagnosis and treatment by eliminating the need to rule out seasonal influenza by testing.

How Does This Apply to You?

In a very simplistic sense, when you avoid those who are ill, you are sequestering yourself. When someone coughs on you and you avoid the newborn baby in your house until you know if you are going to become ill, you are imposing a self-quarantine. When you are ill yourself and you forbid visits by that newborn, you are imposing a form of isolation on yourself. If there is an ill person in your home, you may be using a combination of these concepts in protecting everyone else from illness. When you are up to date with all the recommended immunizations, you are more likely to be part of the solution instead of part of the problem. Think through how you would handle each of these circumstances in your own home during an outbreak. Your *postures* should take them into account.

Protecting Yourself and Your Family

Having a conceptual framework to use in developing your plans and *postures* is important. It is easy to go astray when trying to do something this new and complicated. I would suggest as a model the way the Occupational Safety and Health Administration (OSHA) approached protecting workers from blood borne pathogens. While rules to protect healthcare workers from infectious disease have long been in place, most other workforce segments have few formal requirements for member protection from biological threats. Look at the OSHA concepts to be considered in designing blood-born-pathogen workplace protections and develop an approach to protecting yourself in your home and in the places community locations you still need to visit.

The OSHA concept is based on leaving as little to chance or human error as possible. Universal precautions are designed to get people in the habit of treating everything as infectious. Engineering controls and work practice controls are used to reduce the risk of becoming infected while working. For example, High-Efficiency Particulate Air (HEPA) filtration in air handlers is used to remove infectious particles from the air in some Emergency Rooms and doctors' office suites. Workplace controls, such as the exclusion of persons with certain illnesses from the workplace, are used to further restrict risk. Health care workers with fever and cough should not be caring for patients. Immunizations may be required for the protection of the worker and for the protection of any clients who may be in the workplace. Flu shots are job requirements in many hospitals, given the risk of influenza to already ill persons. Personal Protective Equipment (PPE) including such gloves, eye protection, masks and gowns are required if the presence of infectious agents is possible, usually in affected patient rooms, and other clinical spaces. Patients in isolation rooms in hospitals are cared for by health care professionals appropriately equipped for the disease of concern. Good personal hygiene is a requirement. Everyone has seen signs in restaurants instructing food workers to wash their hands. Hand washing facilities are outside most patient rooms to reduce the possibility of infectious agents being carried room to room by health care providers. These categories of intervention build upon one another to provide the highest level of protection possible with minimal risk of system failure.

Using the same concepts around you and in your home is a good start on planning your self-protection. The term *posture* will be used to describe the way you would do things for a given situation. As the book progresses, you will think of things you want to consider when deciding on your own *postures*. For example, for one *posture*, one for a Pandemic with an airborne spread agent producing severe illness with multiple deaths in your local jurisdiction, but not your home, you might construct a hierarchy like this:

1. Physical Environment- Doors and windows always closed. Only one door to be used for entry and exit. HEPA filter in furnace. Furnace fan set to run continuously. Wash hamper treated as infectious and washed with hot water, detergent and bleach. Surfaces with frequent skin contact cleaned daily. Plastic liners for trash cans with frequent replacement.

2. Access to Home- Family in residence and trusted group only. Entrance protocol of removing PPE and footwear. Outer clothing removed and placed in wash bag, then hands and any exposed skin or hair washed or

sanitized. Trusted group to follow entrance protocol. No other visitors.

3. Personal status- No immunity because this is a new agent.

4. PPE- Mask outside the home. Gloves, eye shield and hand sanitizer carried and used as needed.

5. Venturing out- Food shopping, medical and other essentials only. No work, school, soccer or bridge.

6. Other policies- No unmasked contact outside the home. Exception is home of dad's mother and father as long as neither becomes ill and the household follows the same protocols. Children not to leave home unaccompanied.

The example above is only illustrative. You are unlikely to ever need to face this extreme example. It was written to show how safety of the physical space, and protections such as immunization that do not require further action would be the first line of defense. Universal precautions are taken outside the safety of the home. Next, PPE provides protection when exposure is possible. Finally, policies are devised to make sure the right things are done at the right time. Few situations would require this strict a *posture*.

Personal Protective Equipment

What does the well-dressed person wear, and when? The right outfit for the event. You don't want to under dress, but you don't want to overdress. It is through thinking all of this through, then maintaining an awareness that you will know what is right for you. For 90% of us, having a hand sanitizer and a good mask and glove choice on hand will be enough. The rest of the options are being covered so that the 10% that really need more have some help choosing.

It is easy to say "Personal Protective Equipment" or "PPE", but what items are important for you to have and to know how to use properly? Here are some of the options. It is not an exclusive list, and opinions will vary about what should be used when and where. When in doubt, my own advice hierarchy is Centers for Disease Control (Or

World Health Organization for non-U.S. areas), State Health Department, Local Health Department, my own physician. The governmental agencies all have websites and numbers to call for advice.

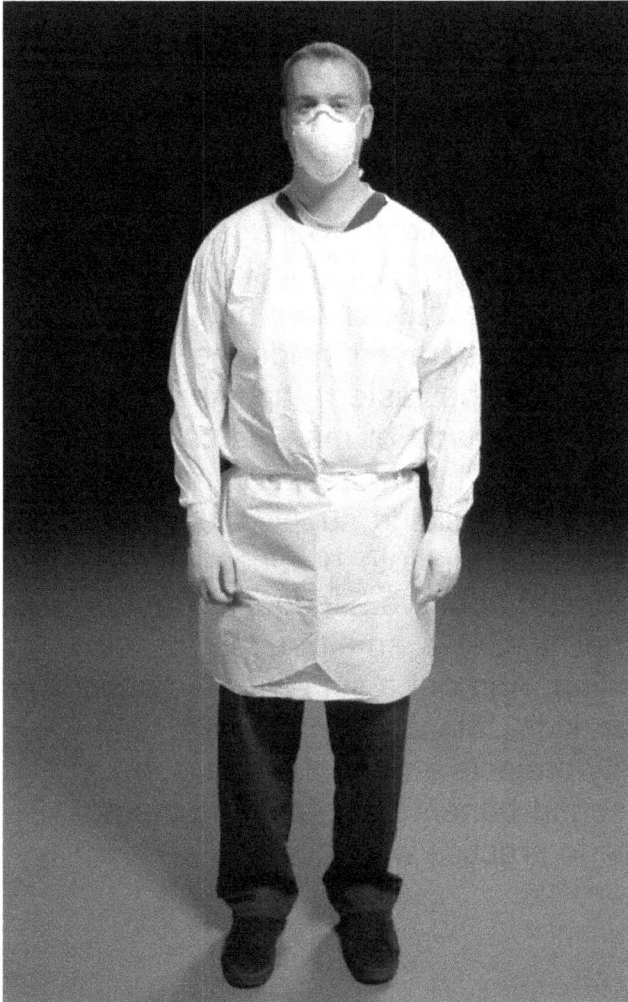

1. Mask

First and foremost, you need a mask that will
keep infection out, fits well, and can be worn

for long periods of time. The **quality** of mask you need for an airborne spread agent is the N-95. It should fit well enough that nothing leaks around the edges. Consider a health care worker being fitted for an N-95 to wear when working with infectious tuberculosis patients. After putting on the mask, a hood would be placed over his or her head, and saccharine would be sprayed inside the hood. If saccharine could be tasted, the mask did not fit properly. This type of mask is called a respirator. If you don't want to spend medical supply prices, try a building supply store. If it is NIOSH (National Institute of Occupational Safety and Health) approved, it doesn't matter where you get it. Get a small supply of the size that fits you. And get a supply of the size that fits your kids. Since you can also use them for dusty projects around the house, you can get a second benefit out of having them, and a chance to practice with them.

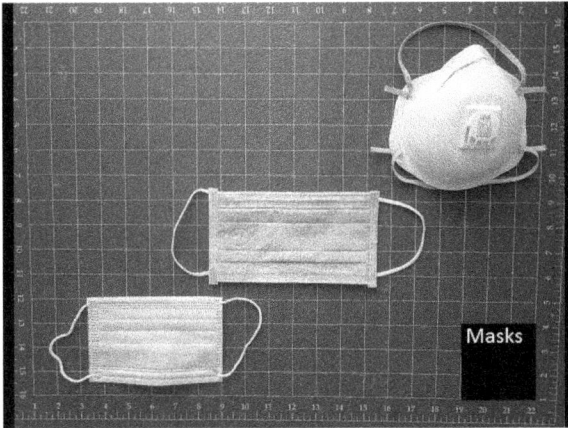

The picture above shows three masks. The one on the lower left is to keep infection IN. If you are sick, you don't want to expose anyone else. If you are sick and use the N-95, every cough will go out the valve, and you waste money. The mask in the center is one that is impregnated with materials designed to kill several viruses. It is a surgical mask, not an N-95. The N-95 on the right is the gold standard.

Not everyone can stand to wear masks for long periods without a sense of claustrophobia. Try one for half a day before you decide what to get. Other devices are far more expensive. There are full face shields with hoods that provide air-tight seals. They usually have small pumps with HEPA filters that continually create a slight over-pressure in the hood. They are called Powered Air Purifying Respirators or "PAPR's." Adult size powered air purifying respirators cost from $400 to $1500 as of this writing.

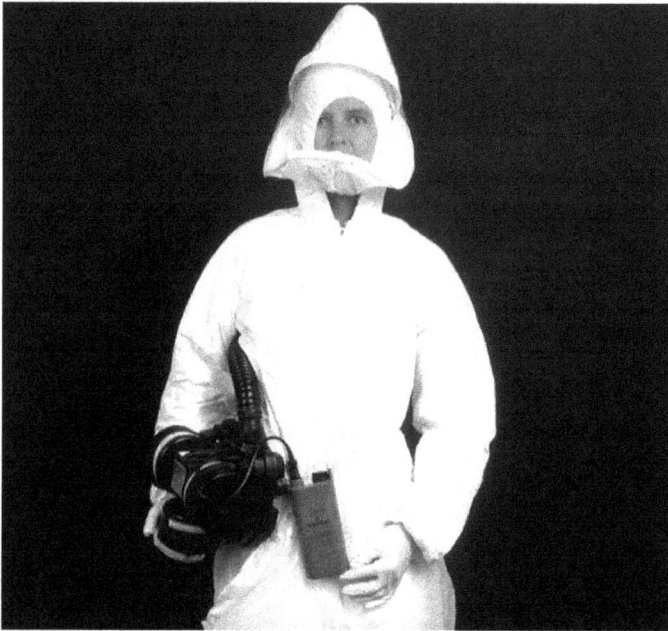

They have the advantages of also protecting the eyes, protecting against splashes, are more comfortable to wear continuously, can be worn by men with facial hair, and protect prescription eyewear from contamination.

Some similar devices are designed for children and even infants. Since these also take batteries and special filter canisters, they would rarely be the option of choice outside of a health care or emergency response setting. You should consult with Public Health or your health care provider before investing in something this expensive and complicated.

2. Gloves

In two of the pictures above, medical quality gloves are being worn. You can use cheaper exam gloves or utility gloves for most things. If you are caring for an ill person, make sure you use a style and quality appropriate for what you are doing. If you are doing things that might puncture your gloves, use the thicker blue "P2" or equivalent. Re-using gloves is not recommended.

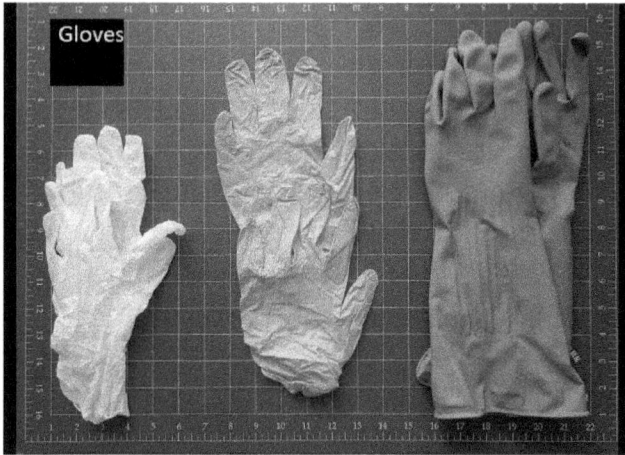

Gloves

The gloves shown above left are latex-free vinyl medical exam quality gloves. They would cover everything but puncture prone situations, but they tend to tear easily. The blue gloves in the center are nitrile-based gloves as you would get at a building supply store. The purple gloves on the right are heavy duty kitchen gloves. While not recommended for patient care, they have the advantage of being washable and hard to tear, and in a long running event you might be happy to have a pair.

You do not need gloves for most activities if you use hand sanitizer or wash your hands frequently. If you are working with materials or people that are clearly contaminated, gloves give you a way to avoid a long and careful scrub after contact. You also avoid worrying about whether you had cuts on your hands or remembered to wash your hands, or whether you washed them enough. If you tend to touch your face or lips or rub your eyes often, you are at risk for infecting yourself. If you have trouble breaking the habit, you might try wearing gloves for a while to help you remember to avoid the habit.

3. Face shield

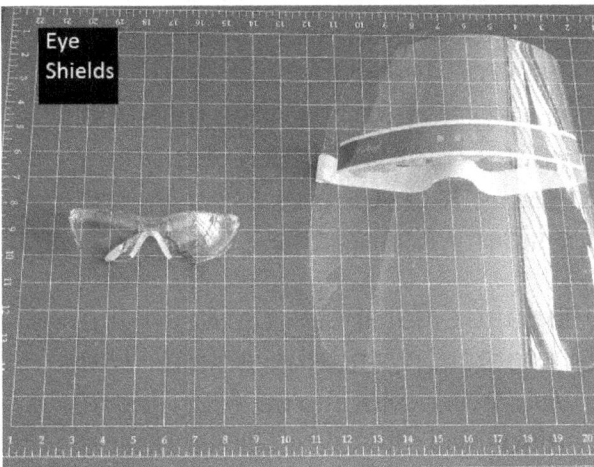

A face shield or eye shield is now worn by many dentists because of the spray they can get in the face. Even when masked, many agents can enter through your eyes if splashed or sprayed in. If you are in a public space where there is coughing and sneezing around you, remember that agents might enter through your eyes if someone coughs or sneezes in your face. Only you can evaluate your surroundings and decide what is right for you. Certain kinds of goggles are now available to be used instead. Both shields and goggles are more convenient and cheaper than a PAPR. Eyeglasses with side shields are an alternative to shields and goggles.

If you are caring for someone who coughs, and can be face to face when they cough, you should wear one or the other. If you are caring for a friend or loved one that needs a lot of hugs to make up for what they are going through, you may be face-to-face enough that you want to consider wearing one.

There are important differences between the eyeglass style protection and the shield. The shield covers you from exposures from more directions. It also will fit over prescription glasses, which usually don't provide adequate protection alone. The glasses style, on the other hand, can easily be carried. Most other situations outside of the workplace should not require either a shield or the glasses style protection. If you are not sure what you may have to deal with, having this kind of protection in your stock is a good idea. If you wind up coming up with *postures* that include them, get them.

4. Gown and booties

These are designed to protect your street clothes from contamination when you have enough exposure to splashes, sprays and puddles on the floor to worry about carrying the agent home on your clothes. At home, you would only consider them if providing care to an ill person and wearing them was part of the Public Health recommendation for the agent. For some agents, not having a gown and getting splashed means you may immediately need to change and launder your clothes, and scrub down. If you expect to be providing care for an ill person with a lot of coughing, sneezing or secretions, having a supply of disposables might be good.

5. Hand sanitizer

There are many brands and sizes of hand sanitizer. The best one is the one you have with you all the time. A small enough bottle to carry is more likely to be in your pocket or purse. Have larger bottles strategically placed around the home and workplace. Make sure the outside of the bottle and the pump for larger bottles are kept clean. Hand sanitizer does not replace a good hand-washing habit. It simply gives you an option when a sink and soap are not convenient.

Summary

What you need to pre-stock depends upon what you see as your roles. Your workplace should provide proper PPE for your job needs. You need to provide for your needs at home, and for getting to and from work. At a minimum, you should have masks and gloves in your more protective **postures**. As you think through the other issues brought up through the book, you will decide whether you need more.

Your Personal Spaces

Remember our examples focus on the highest risk situations, not the most likely ones. If you are protecting yourself and your family from an outbreak in your community, the most important thing to learn first is how is it spread?

How Is It Spreading

For this discussion, a person to person spread scenario is assumed. The current coronavirus epidemic is showing rapid person to person spread.

Airborne spread is where infectious particles can hang in the air and move with air currents. Infectious particles can hang in the air for significant periods. Measles and Smallpox spread this way. There are examples of patients coming to a doctor's office with measles, leaving after being seen, then another person arriving and becoming ill by inhaling infectious particles still in the air long after the first patient left. Few agents spread this efficiently, so don't over-prepare.

Droplet spread is where infectious particles are carried by droplets in the air. Larger droplets tend to fall from the air quickly, limiting the circumstances under which you could be infected. Influenza is spread by droplets that tend to fall out of the air quickly.

A six-foot separation distance from an infected person is usually thought adequate.

Airborne spread is more serious in most environments than droplet spread. Coughing and sneezing can spread infectious particles for both types of disease, but your **posture** should be more protective for an airborne disease than one spread by droplets. You should pick the **posture** that will let you protect yourself in the way most appropriate for each type of transmission and for each specific disease. Public Health will provide guidance on what you need to consider in adjusting your **posture**.

Agents spread either by airborne or droplet mechanisms may also be deposited upon hands, clothing or other surfaces, and be picked up by and infect others from there. This is dependent upon agent characteristics and elapsed time since deposition. Good hand hygiene is even more important where this is a possibility.

In the Coronavirus outbreak, persons have been infected by what appears to be leaking sanitary fixtures and pipes that cause some airborne spread.

Your personal space

Start with your own personal space. Grandmother was right: You should eat properly, get enough rest, cough and sneeze into a handkerchief, and stay away from sick people. Most of our worlds have changed too much to live exactly as she recommended, but the principles are unchanged.

Good personal health helps minimize the impact of illness. The very old and the very young, those with chronic disease, and those with compromised immune systems all tend to have worse outcomes from infections than those with good health. Stress, poor nutrition, sleep deprivation and lack of good social support systems have all been shown to affect the immune system. If you are not in good health, take extra measures to minimize the risk of becoming infected. Avoiding those who are ill and avoiding crowds will reduce exposures. Getting all appropriate available immunizations, and if advised by Public Health taking prophylactic medications, may block infection if you are exposed. If you have significant risk factors because of your health, consult with your caregiver or the Health Department for general guidance now, and for specific suggestions should an outbreak occur.

Fastidious personal hygiene helps protect you and helps protect those around you. Wash your hands frequently, and then be careful what you touch afterwards. Do you grab the knob of the restaurant's bathroom door after washing your hands? The person leaving just ahead of you may have sneezed into his or her hands and then gripped the knob when exiting without washing. If the door swings inward, use the paper towel you used to dry your hands as a door opening aid. When you are outside the bathroom sanitize your hands. Did you sanitize hour hands after reading the menu? How clean is the knob on your bathroom door at home? What might family members or guests have brought to your home from the outside, and deposited on that doorknob? Clean common contact points like doorknobs, faucets, refrigerator door handles and cabinet knobs frequently.

Carry a bottle of hand sanitizer and use it often. Grocery cart handles harbor organisms. Clean them before use if you can. Be aware of the things you touch in public, and decide which to avoid, and when to clean your hands after an unavoidable contact. When severe illness is in the community, maintain your personal space as best you can. Consider using the "SARS Handshake"

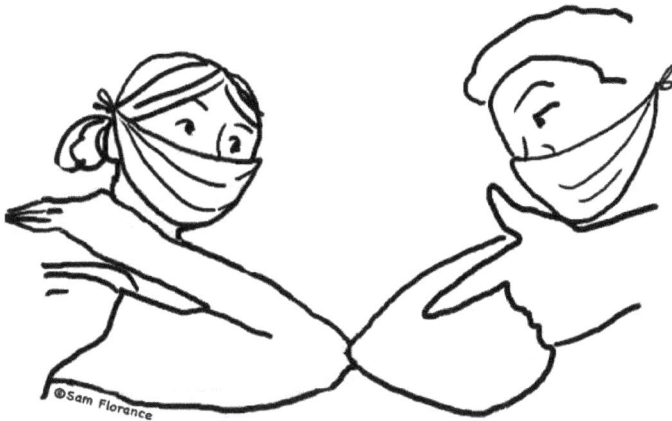

"SARS Handshake"

when greeting people. Bumping elbows is safer than shaking hands if you must touch when greeting someone during an outbreak. Hopefully both of you will bump with the right elbow and reserve the left elbow for the control of sudden coughs or sneezes. Any other habit will mean bumping a contaminated elbow against a clean one, with potential for facilitating spread. Shaking hands with someone who has just sneezed into their own hand is risky. It is too easy to then touch your eye, mouth or in some other way introduce the infectious agent into your body. If you do have to shake hands, use your hand sanitizer immediately after, and offer it to the person you greeted. The single most effective weapon against gastrointestinal disease in U.S. troops in Iraq was good hand hygiene. Hand washing stations were present at the door to every dining facility, and hand sanitizer was at every "porta-potty". Troops quickly learned to be clean or be ill. One reporter was so impressed by everyone lining up to wash before eating that he reported on it in his article!

If you have a sneeze or cough, be conscious of where infectious particles might be going. Direct an unexpected, uncontrollable cough or sneeze into your elbow, not your hand. If you must use your hand, use a handkerchief or tissue if possible, but change it often. Dispose of paper tissues properly and wash your hands or use hand sanitizer before touching anything else.

Make sure your immunizations, particularly for Influenza, are up to date. Many people avoid flu shots because they are afraid the shot itself will make them ill, because they do not believe in shots for personal or religious reasons, or because of cost. In planning for Pandemic Influenza, there was concern that if overwhelming numbers of persons came to the Emergency Room with symptoms of Influenza, the time and resources it would take to differentiate between seasonal Influenza and Pandemic Influenza would contribute to system overload and possible system breakdown, with attendant increased illness and death. A person with up-to-date Influenza immunization could be presumed to have Pandemic Influenza and be treated immediately, while an unimmunized person would require testing to determine which influenza was present and might have treatment delayed if resources were scarce. Since many treatments have potential side effects and adverse consequences, targeted treatment is preferred to presumptive treatment. Which person would you rather be? The person treated immediately, or the delayed person? As this is being written, there are reports of pertussis outbreaks, in some cases involving pertussis variants more resistant to existing antibodies. In the 1990's, a region which allowed childhood immunizations to languish experienced over 50,000 cases of Diphtheria in one year.

FIGURE 1. Number of reported cases of diphtheria — New Independent States of the former Soviet Union, 1965–1995

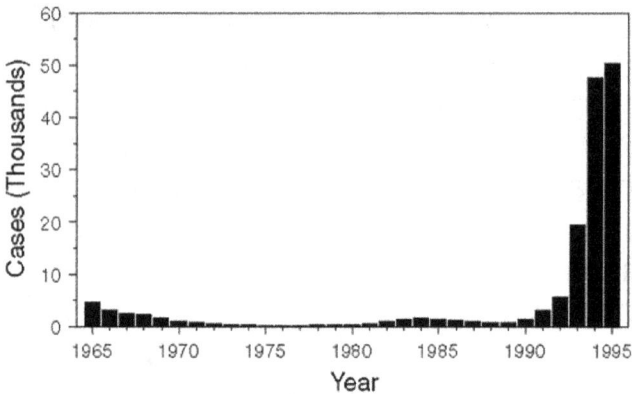

"Herd immunity" is the concept that by having most of the herd immune, the few who are not immune can be shielded from exposure to the disease. It is a balance of the risk of relatively mild adverse reactions in the many against the risk of severe disease in the few. Infants and others with less effective immune systems can have far more serious cases. Antimicrobial prophylaxis for Meningococcal meningitis isn't administered to protect the people receiving it, but rather to protect infants they may be in contact with. This is another case where herd immunity concepts are used to protect those more at risk. Persons who avoid recommended immunization for themselves or their children are weakening the protection for themselves and for the community in general.

If you still aren't convinced, consider the evidence of the Middle School and Measles in the Schools (presented later) outbreaks presented in this book. The agent in the Middle School outbreak appeared to affect one third of the students in the school. Measles affected about 110 students in school populations totaling over 30,000 students. We had no control option for the Middle School gastroenteritis outbreak but to close the school. Updated immunizations were used to stop the measles outbreaks in each school affected without closing the school. This approach prevented measles from being spread to other schools in most cases. The big difference was the very high-level immunity against measles in school populations because of immunizations. What could have happened in the community had it been an agent as infectious as measles, and causing as severe an illness, but one for which no one had immunity? Be part of the solution, not part of the problem. Get all recommended immunizations not medically contraindicated for you. The control of the coronavirus outbreak to date has bought some time to develop a vaccine. If the coronavirus becomes endemic in the U.S. an effective vaccine will be critical to controlling the morbidity and mortality. In such a situation, becoming immunized is your best protection.

Cameo-

Measles and Immune Compromise

During the measles outbreak, it was recognized that there were persons with weakened immune systems in our community who might have bad outcomes if they were exposed to a case of measles. Included were persons with cancer or who were on anti-cancer drugs, persons with

HIV, and persons with organ transplants. We elected to try to notify every person, caregiver or registry that might know of someone at risk. We were told of at least one person who was hospitalized and given intravenous immune globulin because of their risk should they catch measles.

When the swine flu vaccine was distributed a few years ago, the Centers for Disease Control called persons who had experienced Guillain-Barre Syndrome, and recommended they NOT take the vaccine.

In some cases, those contraindications may entail other limitations or treatments for you unneeded by others in the community. Consult with your physician before declining a recommended immunization. Think very carefully before turning down a recommended immunization on purely philosophical or religious grounds.

Your Home-Your Sanctuary or Enclave

You need a place you feel safe. What better place than your home-the place you sleep at night. If you are fearful when you try to sleep, you will not get good rest. Having a sense of safety there, where you spend more time than anywhere else, will give you a feeling of sanctuary. Making sure your home gives you that sense of freedom from risk will be a big step in protecting you both from the risk of illness and from the risk of terror. Awareness of the attributes of the agent causing the outbreak is central to being able to decide what you need to do to feel safe when you are there. Will your space keep out the agent? If you live in a single-family home, the chances an agent will come in with the evening breeze is miniscule. If you live in an apartment with shared air handlers, common hallways and entryways, or elevators, more investigation is needed. Do you live alone, or with others? If you share your living space, can others bring the agent in with them? Again, more investigation is needed. Do you have to go out regularly, such as to work, school, or just to shop? If so, you need to plan your habits around not bringing the agent in yourself.

Be aware of how your living space is heated or cooled. If forced air is used, consider upgrading the filter. A High Efficiency Particulate Air (HEPA) filter will remove most infectious agents, and over time will clear your homes air of any agents that enter. Since these filters tend to be more expensive, unless you need them to control allergens or for some other purpose, have them available but only put them in the air handler when there is an outbreak in the community. If used during an outbreak, treat them as infectious after use and dispose of them properly. Allowing more uncontaminated fresh air into your living space if you cannot filter your air would help dilute those infectious agents that might enter with a visitor.

Keeping your home clean is crucial, particularly if the agent is one that can be infectious if picked up from a surface. Doorknobs are common places for these agents to reside. Just the act of opening your own door to go in can contaminate your hands if an ill person tried the knob earlier. If you are using hand sanitizer regularly, you have one level of protection. If you frequently clean the surfaces in your home, those agents deposited when cough and sneeze aerosols fall from the air can be controlled, and you have a higher level of protection. Do you need a way to clean footwear upon entry? Should all footwear be left at the door? A safe portal of entry is important.

Look at routes of entry. Do you live in a multi-family space? Do you walk down a hallway that might not be agent free? Do you have to use an elevator or stairwell? Elevators are tight spaces often densely packed with people. One cough or sneeze could expose several other people. Consider wearing a mask if illness is in the building and you cannot avoid the elevator. If you are ill yourself, it is particularly important to wear a mask to avoid exposing others. Depending upon the agent involved, you may wish to carefully remove and launder your outside layer each time you re-enter your "sanctuary". Another agent attribute you should try to know is whether you can, in fact, become infected if the agent gets on your clothes. For many agents, this is not a concern, so a lot of peace of mind will be easily obtained with awareness.

You have less control if you share your space with one or more persons who go out regularly. Make sure whatever re-entry procedures you devise are agreed upon and used consistently by all who come into your space. Laundry collection and washing and the detergents used may need to be considered. Planning how to handle the situation when one or more ill persons share your space will be discussed later.

Not all outbreaks are spread by person-to-person exposures. Foodborne and waterborne diseases frequently cause outbreaks. West Nile Virus is spread by mosquitos, and first came to attention as an outbreak. The Zika virus is a more recent virus spread by mosquitos. The rabies epizootic that spread through the Mid-Atlantic states thirty-five years ago was mostly spread by racoons and exposed several people to rabies. Making your home safe from these types of illnesses is straightforward and should be on your check list of tasks.

Feeding yourself

In a serious Pandemic, eating properly may take extra thought. Do you eat out twice a day? Are you the Take-Out King? A sit-down meal at a restaurant may be risky. You would be in a crowded place with your mask off. If you use the salad bar you would be using utensils handled by many other people, and food an ill person might have coughed or sneezed upon. Will you be able to get everything you need at the grocery? If society falters, shopping may be problematic. It may be that your favorite restaurant will convert to take out, or even delivery assisted dining. If there is nothing in your locality Emergency Response Plan to give you comfort on the question, can you take the lead with the restaurant of your choice, or the restaurant community in general? There are many ways nutrition can be maintained, including stocks of "emergency" food. Only you can decide what is best for you, and how to arrange it.

Infants as a special case

Remember that infants do not have a fully functional immune system yet. Even a nursing mother may not be able to protect her infant until she builds immunity herself. Even then, depending on the pandemic agent, it may not be certain protection. Infection control masks are too large for infants. There are resuscitation masks sized for infants, but they won't help you here. Unfortunately, this suggests two limitations you must consider. You cannot safely take an infant out if the process of getting out or the situation at your destination can cause a risk of exposure. Neither can you have anyone come in your house who could expose your infant. It would be very difficult to maintain a "clean room" for your infant if someone in the house was ill. If you have an infant in your household, plan for its safety carefully.

Venturing Out

This book is not about cowering in your home in fear. It is about how you can protect yourself while doing what needs to be done. Groceries need to be obtained, work needs to be done, and school may be in session. You may need to shop for someone who is bedridden. There are endless scenarios. You should consider each reason for leaving your home. For most outbreaks, no changes at all are needed. For those few where Public Health officials recommend reduced public interaction, each type of need should be considered, and a plan made. You can get gasoline for the car without getting close to another person. Getting your hair cut puts you up close to someone with a lot of interaction with other people.

If you live in a multiple family dwelling, the first changes you may have to make may start at your front door. Getting to the street may entail both corridors and an elevator or stairs. Assess the conditions you will encounter getting to the street during an outbreak. If you frequently encounter other people as you exit, you may need to mask during periods when people in the building are ill. If the agent is airborne, even visitors can leave infectious particles in the air. Be aware and assess the building's situation frequently. If you pass people who are actively coughing and sneezing, particularly with poor control of their secretions, even eye protection may be warranted.

Using public transportation has a different set of risks during an outbreak. In a cab, you are only exposed to the driver. In a packed subway during rush hour, the risk of infection is increased if someone coughs or sneezes. Look at each mode of transportation you use. Be aware of the status of the outbreak. Decide daily, if needed, what your *posture* will be. It may be that all you will ever need is a handkerchief in your pocket or purse to hold over your mouth and nose while you breathe if you pass closely to a coughing person. On the other hand, there may be times when high efficiency masks are recommended by Public Health officials. When official recommendations are made, follow them or be even more stringent. Or plan on becoming ill.

Remember the SARS handshake? Most grocery stores now position containers of wipes near the grocery cart pick up point. Wipe your cart handle before you start shopping. Do you need to use public toilets?

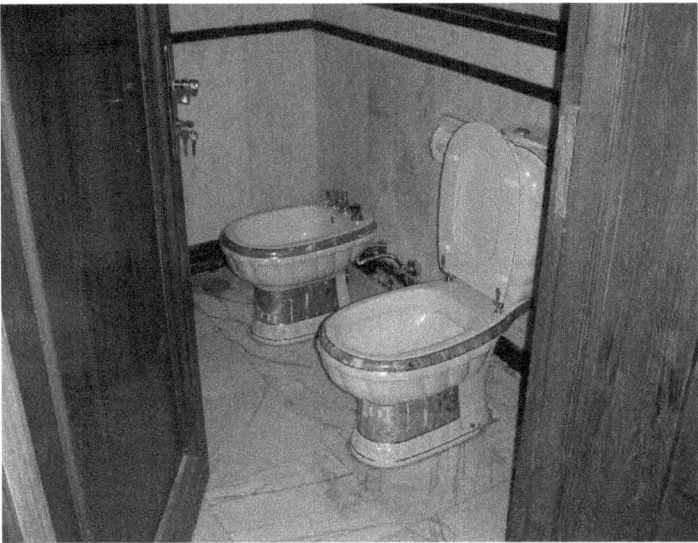

Try to use only those with doors which open out, and which are held shut by springs, not knobs, so you don't have to re-contaminate your hands after washing them by opening the door. If you must use your hands to open the door, use the paper towel you used to dry your hands to insulate your hands from the door while opening it. Drop the paper towel in the waste basket as you leave. Many thoughtful managers now leave a trash container right at the door to facilitate this. If the restroom has no paper towels, use your hand sanitizer after exiting.

Where are you going and how long will you be there? When you are just making short visits to places, maintaining whatever protective posture you deem to be needed is simple. When you are going to be at work, school or other places and interact for extended periods with other people, the problem is more complex. These issues will be addressed as community interactions later.

Coming home again takes some thought. Don't bring the agent into your sanctuary. From your awareness of the properties of the agent causing the outbreak you will know how stringent your measures should be. How much clean up, clothing change, foot gear cleaning and other measures, if any, are to be accomplished each time you re-enter your home? Being ritual bound about this or having and using a checklist will stand you in good stead. The last thing you want to do is remember later the important step you missed. Once you are safely in your home again, that sense of sanctuary should return.

Culture Shock and Self Protection

Without a doubt, learning new habits, adopting protective behaviors and changing the ways you interact with others will engender a sense of culture shock. For instance, your habit may be to give old friends a hug and a kiss on meeting. If you go to stay with family members who live in a relatively unaffected area, remember that with many infectious agents the elderly are at more risk, and you may be unintentionally bringing the agent with you.

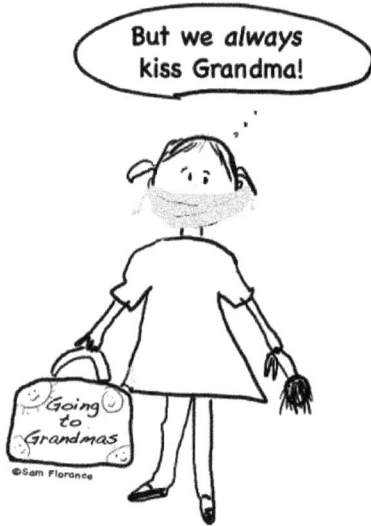

During an outbreak, you may sense they are ill, and you will want to hold back, but are fearful of the hurt they would feel. On the other hand, if you have a feeling of being ill, you won't want to expose them. Thinking through how you might have to change your social habits is important. You are part of many communities, each with its own rules. Some of those rules might have to be changed, ignored, or broken for the best of all concerned. You may feel strange or be chided for taking the precautions you have deemed right for you. Do not be peer-pressured into unsafe behaviors. If you know what you should do in a circumstance, do it and be part of the solution. Take other persons efforts to dissuade you from doing the right thing as teaching opportunities to try to educate them about the risks they are taking.

Even summer camps and retreats can experience disease outbreaks. Refugee camps have more significant risks, and experience difficult situations as a rule. They can also impose a significant culture shock on both residents and staff.

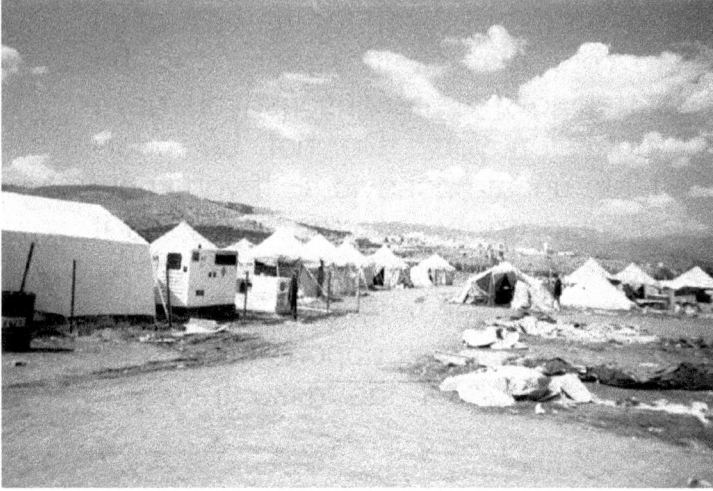

Terror Is a State of Mind!

Terror comes in many forms. Remember the sniper in the National Capitol Region? Have you experienced a "near shot without result" (Winston Churchill) in war? Do you like thrillers at the movies or on TV? Have you experienced a life-threatening event where your adrenaline surged, and your pulse bounded? Do you fear tax-day, a big exam, or a job interview? Most people can think of stressful times or events that induced physiological responses. At the extreme, these responses can be paralyzing. The fear can be so intense that panic or inability to respond overwhelms the person involved, and the person responds in a way they may regret later. Even outbreaks of disease can inspire fear. Courage is not being without fear, it is being able to perform well while fearful. Terror is a state of mind where the fear rules.

Cameo-

5 cases of Anthrax, 3 million cases of terror

As the Anthrax incident in the Washington Metropolitan Area unfolded, there were many people who were fearful that they had been infected and came to the Emergency Room or their physician's office seeking testing, treatment, prophylaxis, or all three. Even though much information was being made available through the media, no one seemed to be convinced by it. There were in fact many people who had been in workplaces contaminated with Anthrax spores, or who were contaminated or exposed in some way. They needed to be questioned, then tested and treated or given antibiotic prophylaxis depending upon their own circumstance. Most of these persons were identified through workplace investigations. The overlap of the various groups with exposure, symptoms, fear without exposure and illness is shown below. The numbers are all estimates.

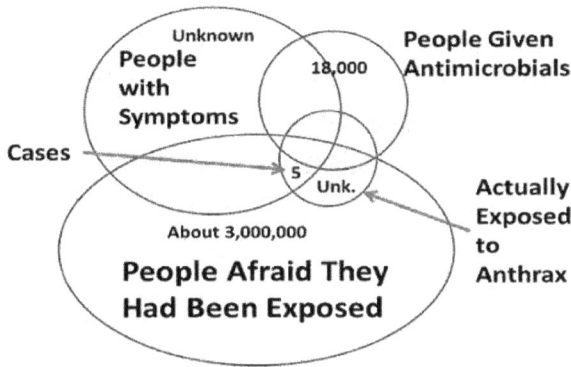

Unknown
People with Symptoms

People Given Antimicrobials

18,000

Cases

5
Unk.

Actually Exposed to Anthrax

About 3,000,000

People Afraid They Had Been Exposed

To ensure that everyone who thought they might have been exposed could walk in for evaluation, clinics were set up across the region to distribute antibiotics. The clinics created an access point outside hospitals, no one had to be turned away, and the almost overwhelming workload being seen in Emergency Rooms was reduced significantly. It was never clear just how many people were exposed, but about 18,000 persons received prophylactic antibiotics.

This number was far larger than the number of people really exposed, but there was no way to definitively show freedom from exposure, so it was hard to limit the number provided prophylaxis without putting some people at risk of Anthrax. Since many people failed to complete the course of antibiotics, it is probable that the side effects of the medications caused some to re-evaluate the probability that they had been exposed and decide they had not been. Not all patients with symptoms had symptoms of Anthrax. Not everyone who was fearful had symptoms or had been exposed. It is simplistic to say that there were 5 cases of Anthrax and 3 million cases of terror, but that is what it seemed like to those trying to manage a difficult situation. There were NO cases that occurred because of failure to provide prophylactic antibiotics.

This is not to ascribe fault to those who were worried but unexposed. Many people did not have a way to assure themselves that they were unexposed. It was a truly frightening time for many people. With so many people commuting by bus and Metro (subway), no one could be sure in their own mind that they had not brushed up against someone with contaminated clothing. Some of the persons who were worried enough to come forward probably *had* been exposed. Fortunately, none developed Anthrax. This is a clear message that preparation by each person for the arrival of community-acquired-infections of resistant organisms can help reduce fear and anxiety when one occurs. By being prepared, knowledge, not fear, can guide your actions.

Fear of exposure to Anthrax by mail was also widespread. Every letter was suspected as having been in the same mail bag as one of the Anthrax letters. Calls to 911 by worried mail recipients were frequent. But the cartoon by Brian Duffy shown below captures for me the spirit of people in the U.S. at that time. Battered by the 9/11/2001 attacks followed by the Anthrax letters, we were still coping, still going to live our lives undaunted, and without losing our sense of humor.

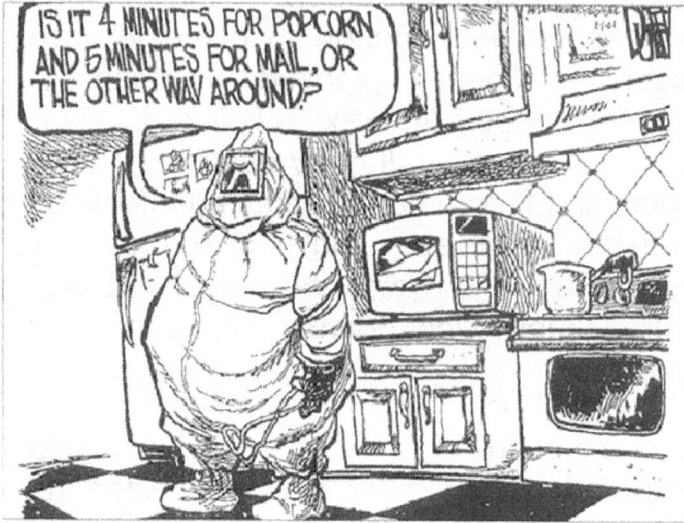

For me this cartoon was a tension reliever, and a reminder that terror is a state of mind we can deal with.

Cameo-

Responding to the Anthrax letter call to 911

Many, many calls were responded to by local agencies. These all proved to be false alarms but showed again how pervasive fear can become when people are not comfortable with the information available to them about their own risk. The County Hazardous Materials Officer devised a special Anthrax letter investigation tool, shown below.

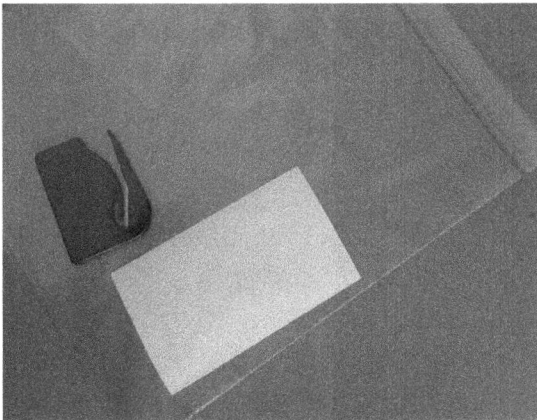

When a call came to the 911 center from someone fearful, thinking they had been exposed by a letter, a police officer, not a rescue squad, was dispatched. The officer would be dressed in daily uniform, not protective equipment. That would set the tone. The officer would put the letter inside the zip lock bag and open it with the letter opener while the bag was sealed. The person would be asked if they were a

target, if the letter was a threat, if the letter contained an unexpected material, if there was an exposure, and if there were symptoms. An examination of the contents was often followed by something like this:
 Officer: "Ma'am, you are a retired teacher. It is not likely you were a target. This is your phone bill. It may seem threatening, but it is not the kind of threat we mean. The powder on it is a powder that is generated by the printing process. It is not Anthrax." The calm, professional response invariably resolved the issue, and no Emergency Room visit was made. Out of about 400 letters, 6 were tested, but not one was contaminated. No one chose to go to the Emergency Room, and no one became ill from Anthrax. A well designed response plan can go a long way towards relieving the anxiety of the public it serves.

Thinking through how you would respond ahead of time will make it easier for you to know what to do if the time should ever come when you need to decide whether you are at risk. Time and subconscious contemplation will help you get from intellectual understanding to emotional acceptance and will make terror much less likely. It would be hard not to be fearful in many situations, but if you can keep the fear under control, you will be far better off.

By thinking out the issues ahead of time, you will also come to a set of personal values that will help you get through an event. You may even find that you will develop a personal credibility in some areas, and that you yourself can become a calming influence and a voice of reason in some situations unimaginable to you today. Just as fear can be infectious, so can courage and calmness. People will follow an example they respect.

"A healthy attitude is contagious but don't wait to catch it from others. Be a carrier"- Tom Stoppard

Cameo-

Meningococcal Meningitis Outbreak?

One year there was a case of Meningococcal meningitis in a college student in Maryland. This is a very severe, often fatal type of meningitis. A week later, there was another case in a schoolteacher

139

in our community. This type of meningitis was uncommon in our community but did occur from time to time. Two cases were unusual enough to get the attention of the TV news community. By the time they called we had done our homework and had found the two cases to be totally unrelated. Though unexpected, two cases in the area a week apart were not improbable. When the TV crews arrived, the stress the reporters felt was evident. During the taping of a segment for the evening news, you could see the stress bleed off as the situation was described and questions were answered authoritatively and calmly. When the segments aired that night, the tone was to calm the community, not to inflame.

Credibility is a Public Health Officer's stock in trade. When you have a reputation for honesty and correctness, people will listen. When you have a responsible news media, and fortunately we did, the right message will get out and be a great service in reducing unnecessary fear. Prior thoughtful consideration and emotional acceptance will help you develop the values, standards and behaviors you need, and will help you live them every day, not just espouse them. This will greatly improve your situation should an event occur. Be aware, be calm and authoritative and be honest. You will develop that credibility yourself. If the time comes when you are in front of the camera, remember that sensationalism will tend to worsen the fears people already have. Be calm, be correct, and try to be part of the solution.

Postures

Seeing what you have learned

Summarize your understanding of what you have read by defining one or more plans and **postures** that you could implement in a Pandemic. Here are some examples.

1. Situation:

Cases are being seen throughout the community. No school closures or formal social distancing measures have been advised. It is a viral Influenza-like illness of such severity that the Emergency Room in one hospital is on bypass. Nationally, there have been several deaths, mostly in children. This year's Influenza vaccine has been very effective. You received your Influenza immunization 5 weeks ago. You live alone.

a. Plan: Continue normal activities

b. **Posture**:   No extra measures are needed.

2. Situation:

As above, but you have a 3-year-old at home, and neither of you are immunized.

a. Plan: Obtain immunizations immediately. Avoid all unprotected contacts. Close home to visitors. Mask child when away from home. Avoid activities outside the home. Resume normal activities when you are told you are immune by your health care provider or the Health Department.

b. **Posture**: Mask when venturing out. Carry hand sanitizer and use frequently. Re-entry cleaning protocol. HEPA filter in home air handler. Return to baseline when immune.

3. Situation:

As above, but there is no vaccine, and the situation is worsening. Hospital is overloaded, and there have been local fatalities.

a. Plan: Obtain prophylactic antivirals if available. No visitors. The door is not opened for anyone. Deliveries are left outside the door. Upgrade filter in the air handler to HEPA. Masks when going out. Minimize outside contacts. Carry hand sanitizer and use it frequently. Wash clothes on returning home. Sanitize doorknob and high use surfaces frequently. No contacts for child outside the home, including no day care. Telecommute.

b.   *Posture*: Mask when venturing out. Gloves to touch any secretions outside the home. Hand sanitizer carried and used frequently. Re-entry protocol when coming home. No physical contact with persons outside the home. HEPA filter in air handler.

These examples are not intended to be prescriptive of how you would organize your own plan, or what you would do for each situation. They are designed to illustrate the need to have different *postures* for different situations, and facts you might consider when deciding what to do when. Develop and write down a set of *postures* that make sense to you, and that you can adhere to. Once your plans tell you to adopt a particular *posture*, there are no more decisions you must make, and life gets easier. You only need a few, well-defined *postures* from which you can choose the best for a given situation as you develop your plans. If you try to do a plan and unique **posture** for every eventuality, it will be like trying to eat an elephant.

Eating the elephant in small bites

Try to keep things simple. It is hard to follow a complicated scheme. You either need PPE or you don't. If you do, you probably only need to have two options: Mask alone, or mask, eye protection and gloves. In all cases you will be using a lot of hand sanitizer. It is the same with immunizations and antimicrobials. Either they have them, they will get them, or you are on your own. If they have them, until *you* have them you need to protect yourself. The examples below illustrate how you can work to come up with a simple set of rules and **postures**.

1. Availability of immunization:

The worst case is no immunization is available. The best case is you are already immunized with a vaccine known to be very effective.

a. For no vaccine: See 2. below

b. For a vaccine you have just taken: See 2. below. Follow those plans and *postures* until you are immune. You will be told how long that will be when you get the immunization. Once you are immune, plan and *posture* is as for no outbreak.

c. You are known to be immune: Plan and *posture* is as for no outbreak.

2. Mechanism of spread:

The worst-case scenario is an airborne disease that can hang in the air for hours. Prepare first for that. You can then simplify your plans and *postures* for something spread by droplets. For example, if you work in a large office with several other people, and one of them is ill and coughing:

a. For an airborne disease: Your plan would be to wear your PPE or leave the area. Your *posture* for the disease might be mask and eye protection, with gloves if touching other people or potentially contaminated objects.

b. For a droplet spread disease: You might work without PPE and remain in the area if you could always maintain adequate separation. You should keep your desk clean with frequent wiping. Your *posture* would be gloves for surface and personal contact away from your desk. Mask when away from your desk, when working within 6 feet of another person or if people pass closer than that to you while at your desk. In this situation, you don't know for sure everyone will remain unexposed, so you assume anyone could be infectious.

3. Status of Pandemic:

In the next section, **What Should You Do When**, six levels of plan and *posture* are suggested for you to consider. These levels go from **No threat** to **It is in your home**. If you are maintaining awareness, and you find that an outbreak is starting to spread in other countries, find out if a vaccine is available. Getting it before it reaches the U.S. may give you time to build immunity and avoid a lot of difficulty. Otherwise, you may have to start adjusting your plans and *postures* as information about the agent becomes available, as the severity of the Pandemic is determined, and as immunizations and other pharmaceuticals are developed and become available.

If someone is ill in your home, other questions must be asked. If you are immune, you can provide sick care without fear. If you are not immune, you either must adopt a safe *posture* when providing care or have someone else provide it. In addition, your home itself must have a higher *posture* so that the ill person will be adequately isolated from unexposed and unprotected persons.

It still seems like a lot of options, but when you cross off the things that don't apply to you, the problem can be managed. That is also why you want to write your plans out. When the time comes, you only have to pick up your plan and do it.

Don't become complacent

Don't assume that this will all happen in a fast time frame.
Developing and distributing new immunizations is a time-consuming task. Plan for the worst case as outlined above, so that all you must do is ease off on your plans if things go well.

The example just above was work related. You should go through the same thoughts for each community you will be participating in during the Pandemic. You should find that the concepts in your plans and **postures** are consistent, and that you are protecting yourself the same way in every place the chance of exposure is the same.

A side benefit of this planning and preparation is that you can better respond to everyday annoying exposures such as adolescents coughing and sneezing on the bus or the person behind you at the movies coughing on the back of your head. You can choose to use the same concepts to develop a **posture** for everyday use during the cold and flu season.

What Should You Do When?

A question you must always consider is how ready you need to be. Reports of new diseases, unexplained disease clusters of unknown cause and suggestions of impending severe Influenza seasons can keep you anxious. You do not need to wear a mask to the grocery store just now. Maybe asking friends to stay away is a trifle excessive. There will probably never be the kind of Pandemic that people have forecast, but what if....

Do now

There are some prudent steps to take now, so that you can continue your everyday life with few if any changes. Consider some of the suggestions below, and how they would affect your risk of catching everyday illnesses:

1. Look at your personal habits and make adjustments to behaviors that would be important in an event but could also leave you vulnerable to frequent common colds or other maladies.

a. Be fastidious about hand cleanliness. Wash your hands after using the restroom or handling anything likely to be a source of infection. This would include, but is not limited to, shopping carts, subway and bus grab bars, doorknobs, and similar places touched by the public at large. Wash your hands before eating or snacking. If you are constantly touching your face, lips and eyes, try to break yourself of the habit.

b. Carry and use hand sanitizer. It will be handy for the multitude of times you cannot wash your hands at a sink when trying to comply with the previous suggestion.

c. Don't re-contaminate your hands after washing at a public toilet. If the exit has a door that swings in, grasp its handle with the paper towel you used to dry your hands, then dispose of the towel properly. If the toilet is not equipped to let you do this, use your hand sanitizer after you exit.

d. Sanitize your hands after shaking hands. This can be done in an inoffensive way if you practice. The other person may be incubating a cold, and just sneezed into the hand offered.

e. Trap uncontrollable sneezes and coughs in your elbow if you cannot use a tissue or handkerchief. Then sanitize your hands

f. Carry tissues or a handkerchief so that you can trap your own coughs and sneezes, blow your nose, or wipe saliva or other secretions. Dispose of tissues properly, then clean your hands with sanitizer. If you find you are using a handkerchief too frequently, use tissues instead. Don't make a habit of carrying a used handkerchief.

2. Organize your living and workspaces to reduce opportunity for infection.

a. Place tissues at strategic places. Have waste baskets in convenient locations and empty them frequently.

b. Make sure your air handler, if you have one, has a good, clean filter, and change it as recommended. If you can afford to do so, use High Efficiency Particulate Air (HEPA) filters in your air handler all the time. Doing so will also remove allergens and reduce the amount of dust you must clean from your home.

c. Make sure every sink has soap or sanitizer.

d. Evaluate your spaces. Look for "public contact" surfaces where guests and visitors will place their hands. Clean those places regularly, and immediately after a visitor with a cough or cold departs.

e. Make sure you dispose of waste properly. Used tissues and other potentially infectious waste should be placed in tightly closed plastic garbage bags. If someone in the home is coughing or sneezing, plastic-bag used air filters as well. The trash collector doesn't want to get sick either.

3. Conduct yourself as you would wish others to conduct themselves.

a. If you have a cough, cold or other potentially infectious condition, keep your distance from those who cannot afford to be ill. This is not the time to kiss the new grandchild or the older relative with cancer.

b. Always trap your sneezes and coughs, and hand sanitize afterwards. Be careful to dispose of used tissues in a way that someone else will not contact them.

c. If you car-pool or otherwise spend time in confined spaces with others, and become ill, avoid the contacts. At a minimum, make them aware ("folks, I think I'm coming down with a cold") and let them decide what risk they want to take. Wearing a mask while carpooling if you have an upper respiratory illness would be appropriate.

d. Think back on the times someone has coughed on you, or otherwise made you feel at risk, and resolve never to do likewise. Set the example.

4. Develop a stock list of things you would want to have every day, let alone during a Pandemic. The FEMA webpage has a section with recommendations for home stocks for disasters in general. Decide what you want to have for all disasters, and for Pandemics in particular, and keep enough on hand so that you never run out. Then add enough extra so that you don't have to run to the store when Influenza or something worse is in the community and supplies are scarce. Such things might be:

a. Extra soap and hand sanitizer. Stock bottles can be used to refill the bottle in your pocket.

b. Tissues. Boxes for home and office, packs to carry.

c. Masks and gloves are a must. Decide what quality you need and think of how often you will change them given your habits. It is better to have a few extras. You can always rotate stocks by using them during projects or cleaning. Other Personal Protective Equipment (PPE) stocks would depend on what you plan to be doing.

d. Plastic garbage bags to line trash cans so used tissues, etc., don't have to be touched again. A small supply of used plastic shopping bags might be worth keeping on hand for this purpose, but if you use them be careful to over-pack them with a plastic garbage bag before putting them out in the trash.

e. Stock one or two High Efficiency Particulate Air (HEPA) filters for your air handler, if you have one. If you can't afford them, stock spare regular filters.

f. Have a detergent based cleaner to use in cleaning surfaces.

g. Have a supply of chlorine bleach. Diluted 1:100, or 1/4 cup in a gallon of water, it is a good cleaner for surfaces during a Pandemic. It is a known asthma risk, and can be toxic to eyes and skin, so use gloves and other PPE as needed for the situation.

h. If you might be caring for an ill person in your home or enclave during a severe Pandemic, consider having a supply of heavy clear plastic sheeting and duct tape to use in separating the patient space from that used by those who are not ill.

5. Develop your concepts for self-protection and construct plans for how you would deal with a range of possible situations.

a. Include as a minimum six levels of plan and of *posture* for use in a Pandemic.

1). No threat is known. Essentially this is the "do now" level.

2). A Pandemic threat has been identified, but no outbreak has occurred.

3). The Pandemic agent is spreading but is not in the U.S. If you work at an Airport or other port of entry, you might implement the next higher set of plans if the outbreak is in a country that feeds your facility either directly or indirectly.

4). The Pandemic is in the U.S.

5). The Pandemic is in your community.

6). The Pandemic is in your house.

b. Develop a *posture* for each of your levels. For each *posture* consider (at a minimum):

1). How "tight" will you make your home or enclave? Do you upgrade your air filter? Do you restrict entry by others? What are your hygiene measures on re-entry? How do you dispose of used PPE? Do clothes worn outside require laundering?

2). What is your protection level (PPE) when you venture out? Do you mask before exiting because you must transit a hall or elevator? Do you mask while car-pooling or using mass transit? Do you have any activities that require gloves? Do you need a checklist before exiting to make sure you haven't forgotten anything?

3). What changes do you make to activities while out? Do you stop attending group functions? Should you adopt precautions at work, school or other mandated activity because the activity does not have controls that meet your standard? Do you adopt precautions at the grocery because of potential exposure?

4). If someone who is ill will be in your home, do you need to create separate space to protect those who are not ill? This may not be an issue if prophylactic pharmaceuticals or immunizations will be provided in a timely way, but plan for it until you know.

6. Determine what sources of information you will use in deciding which level you should be using. Be specific. That is, will you use a particular news source? Does the Health Department, local jurisdiction, Department of Homeland Security, or some other government agency have a timely web page or other way for you to stay informed? You don't want to respond to scare, you want to respond to RISK.

7. Decide who you will trust. This will be a very difficult and delicate process. Friends and family will be insulted if you do not include them. Make a list of who you will trust. Make a *private* list of those you will NOT trust, and the reason. This way you can make it a teaching moment if the question arises. After all, part of what you want to do is help

everyone else survive too. If you don't write it down, you may have trouble remembering or being able to articulate your reasons when you are under the stress of a Pandemic. No matter how careful you are yourself, if you have unprotected contact with a person you do not trust, you may be reminded by becoming ill of the reason you didn't want to trust them.

When a Pandemic is on the horizon

This is the second level suggested above. A threat has been identified, but no outbreak has occurred. At this point, some information should be available as to the nature of the threat.

1. Review your plans and **postures**. Make any adjustments based upon the nature of the risk. A widespread "a little worse than usual" Influenza prediction might ease the situation for most people, while prediction of another SARS virus might influence you to be more thorough. If it is something *really big*, start thinking in terms of your stricter **postures**.

2. Review your stocks. Make sure you have on hand what you have forecast as needed.

Add anything that might be now considered important. If something big gets to the U.S., the things you have in your plan may suddenly be in short supply.

3. Discuss the situation with your trusted group to make sure you are all on the same page.

When the Pandemic is starting to spread

It is starting to spread but is not in the U.S. yet. At this point, National and International agencies will be working to keep the Pandemic out of the U.S. if possible. The greatest risk is from travelers by air. If someone can enter the U.S. incubating the disease and not be detected, they could arrive at almost any airport in the country in an infectious state, then move on to another. Several airports could be contaminated by a few people this way. People who have contact with travelers who might fit this description should consider adopting their posture for "In the U.S." even before it gets here. For everyone else, awareness is important, but the probability of being the first ill person in your community is low.

1. If you are in a densely populated area with a high level of international travel, you might consider increasing your *posture* level. If you live in the country and have little possibility of being the first in the U.S. to be exposed, adopt whatever posture you planned for this level.

2. Review your plans, *postures* and stocks.

3. Update your awareness of the situation regularly, and adjust plans, *postures* and stocks as needed.

4. Discuss the situation with your trusted group to make sure you are all consistent in your approach.

The Pandemic is in the U.S., but not your community

This could happen if it starts here instead of being imported. There is now a significant potential for this arriving in your community without warning.

1. If you are in frequent contact with others, particularly travelers, consider a higher level of *posture*. Otherwise, implement your plan and *posture* for this level.

2. Conduct your reviews, update your awareness and discussions as above. You may have some time before it appears in your community. Expect your chosen information source(s) to keep you well informed as to local risk and recommended measures.

3. Adjust your plans and postures as needed to comply with any official guidance provided.

4. Coordinate with your trusted group.

The Pandemic is in your community

Implement your plan and *posture* for this level. Depending on the severity of disease caused by the Pandemic agent, you must be zealous in adhering to them.

1. At this time, you should consider everyone you meet to be exposed. The exceptions to this assumption should only include those you trust with your life. Roommates, your spouse,

children and friends all can become exposed accidentally if they are not in an appropriate **posture** for the situation, or otherwise fail to protect themselves for whatever reason. Small children especially need to be made gently aware of the importance of your safety rules. If possible, try to avoid making them feel frightened, mad or overly anxious.

2. Unless you are visiting a trusted enclave, always maintain your posture. Once you are exposed, you are exposed.

3. Maintain the best awareness of the situation you can get. In a Pandemic, sources of information and sources of supply may dwindle.

4. Keep up your own surveillance of those around you. At the first sign that the agent is breaching the walls of your trusted group, you will have to re-evaluate your situation and your plans.

5. If any prophylactic or treatment pharmaceuticals are recommended, obtain them and use them when and if directed. If any additional resources are recommended in

case someone in your home becomes ill, obtain them.

The Pandemic is in your home

If someone in your home is exposed or becomes ill, you must adopt the most stringent measures possible to protect yourself and others.

1. Warn others in your trusted circle. No one needs to be blind-sided. You may have to report the situation to an agency.

2. Implement quarantine and/or isolation as appropriate. Try to limit further exposure in your home. If only an exposure has occurred, and the person is not ill, you may have the option to quarantine at home. If consistent with Public Health guidance, and if the exposed person can be quarantined in a separate space, you have a better opportunity to protect everyone else. If the person is already ill, then depending upon the agent, others in your home may already be exposed. If possible, discuss this with competent authority. This is a situation that requires careful evaluation. Hopefully, your plan and *posture* has allowed for it.

3. Provide sick care to anyone who is ill. Do so in a way that protects you from exposure. You can't help anyone if you are ill yourself. For serious or life-threatening illness, the person should be moved to a health care facility if possible. The local jurisdiction will provide guidance on what should be done.

Protecting Yourself in Your Communities

We are all members of communities. By community we don't just mean the cluster of buildings around your home. The term is being used broadly to include every distinct grouping of people in which you or a family member participates. For this discussion, communities will include families, schools, day care, work, commuting, travel, and any other place where you associate with people. In each community aggregations of people provide opportunities for disease spread. Look at the nature of the membership of each community, the patterns of interaction within the community and the physical environment of the community. Each community you interact with and physical place you visit will need to be considered for its risks to you. Concepts need to be developed for assuring your self-protection with each one.

Cameo-

Communities and Community Spread

The 1988 measles outbreak in our county illustrates many features of outbreaks you should understand. For now, just the spread throughout the county schools will be discussed. Other Cameos will explore other facets of the outbreak. At first there was one case, one school. A week later, there were two cases, each in a different school. The week after, we were up to 4 cases in three different schools. Another week, tens of cases in 8 schools. Then 9 schools. Finally, over 100 cases in 11 schools.

The case plot below shows how the outbreak jumped from school to school. Some jumps were because one child infected a sibling who attended another school, or both were infected by a third person who was not identified. In at least one case, a sports team from one school had an infectious person at a meet, and an infection was passed on to a student at the other school. Other social jumps included boy-girl couples that attended different schools, carpools, and the like. These were not theoretical ways an outbreak could spread, but documented cases identified during the outbreak investigation. Because there were subclinical cases, students were infected by people they did not realize were sick, let alone infectious. The student body overall was highly immunized. It was the very small population with no immunity or waning immunity which was susceptible. Several thousand immunizations were given to under-immunized students during clinics held in the schools. If a clinic was held quickly enough after the first case in the school appeared, there were no further cases.

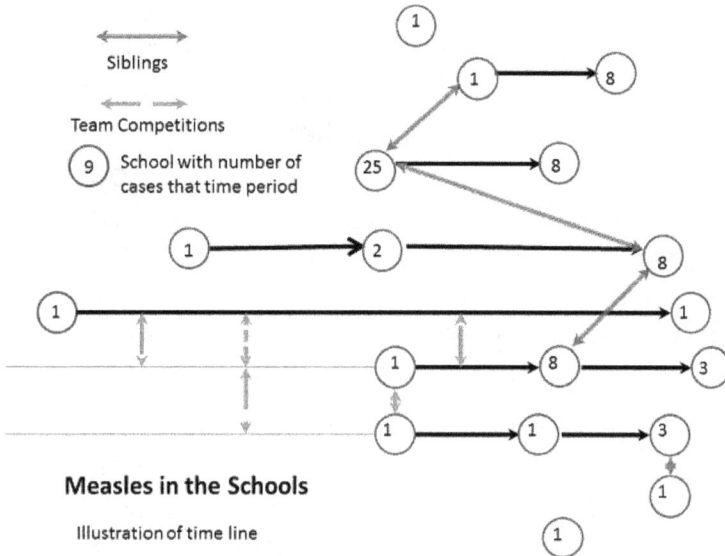

Siblings

Team Competitions

(9) School with number of cases that time period

Measles in the Schools

Illustration of time line

One message here is that you must use extreme care and be exhaustive in considering where you and your family members interact in communities if you want to "sequester" yourself and your family during an outbreak. Not only must you identify all the places of potential risk, but you must decide how you will deal with that risk. Think in terms of changing how you participate and what your personal protective posture will be. Understand your communities, and whether adjustments need to be made to your social and work habits.

Another message here is that an outbreak can easily move from one locality to another as work goes on, as family members visit family, as people vacation, and so on. One of the activities of Public Health is to evaluate each connection between localities and try to minimize the movement of the agent between them. The news occasionally gives accounts of ill persons being removed from airplanes, and once reported on a person who knew he had communicable treatment-resistant tuberculosis and flew on an airline even though he had been counseled to not do so.

The third message here, and the reason I showed the progression over 5 weeks, is that one of the goals of our response to a Pandemic is to slow its spread around the world and across the country to buy time. Each "jump" had to wait for the measles to incubate. If you can slow each "jump" by another incubation period, you have slowed the progress of the Pandemic to half speed. That could be a lot of time bought!

The list of communities considered below is certainly not exhaustive. You must list EVERY community in which you participate and decide what your level of interaction will be with that community during a Pandemic. Just remember that every time you add a community to your list of those you would be involved with during a Pandemic, you increase the possibility that if you became ill while participating in one, you could expose the members of all of the others.

Family

For many persons, family is the most important community. You may only need to consider a nuclear or extended family that resides in your home. If so, your job is a little easier. If you have a family with members that reside in other homes, but with whom you interact constantly, you may have to treat them as an outside community and have different **postures** to use when meeting at your home or theirs.

If there is a dominate family decision maker, that person must be fully on board, and take leadership. Be a leader in helping your family be safe. Be aware of the health status of each person in the family and move quickly to limit spread of infection in your own household if it should appear. Know the guidelines for infection prevention in the community, and make sure everyone in the family who goes out knows and follows those rules. Ask children who have been at school, play or just "out" whether they noticed anyone being ill. Have a daily family activity to go over the family plan, guidelines, and risks and potential exposures incurred that day. Decide ahead of time how you will manage the home if someone were to become exposed or ill, then stick to the plan should it happen.

Your home's environment was briefly discussed earlier. Now look at the group interaction patterns of family residing at home, and the patterns of guests and visitors. Decide what group habits need to be developed or changed, and work with each family member, and the family as a group, to come to whatever agreements and norms are possible. If the nearest ill person is cities away, you have a different need than if the outbreak is in full swing in your local area. Have rules in place for when you want to implement your plans, and to what level of protection.

If there is exposure or illness in your home, can you use tape and plastic sheeting to separate parts of the dwelling to help segregate well persons from the exposed and the ill? Can you provide a means of sequestering bread winners or others who must go out to ensure their continued freedom from illness? Should you provide informal quarantine for a family member who is exposed, while waiting to see if illness occurs? Are you able to provide isolation for one who is ill, provide medical care, and still protect the rest of the family? Are you able to keep a coughing ill person in your house but control the movement of infectious particles throughout the house? Do you have any materials you would need to accomplish this? What about medical supplies, sanitizers and waste disposal? During a Pandemic, many things may become scarce. Decide on a reasonable stock of items you decide would be critical, obtain them now, and keep your stock up to date by using it day to day but replacing it day to day. You might consider developing carry packs with hand sanitizer, handkerchiefs and/or tissues, mask and gloves for each member of the family, with easy refill at home and in the car.

Formally write down your plan and your rules. Make frequent checks, at least until the new habit is well established, to make sure everyone carries their **posture's** supplies each time they leave home. Hold daily family discussions to share information on who in the community is ill, discuss any potential exposures and so forth. The importance of having the family decision maker take the lead in this cannot be overemphasized. The head of the family is often the role model for others in the family, and just by doing the right thing will encourage others to do so as well.

School and work

The most common communities outside the home are work and school. They are also communities likely to have their own rules, rules that may be strictly enforced, yet rules that may or may not fit what must happen during a major outbreak. Both communities are likely to entail frequent near random meetings between people. They are often likely to involve interactions with members of other similar communities. These factors combine to create unavoidable opportunities to meet infectious people. The trick is to develop **postures** that will let you participate as you need to without actually becoming exposed by people with whom you are in contact. You might develop a comfort zone around safety in your office or classroom itself. Do your homework first, and make sure the environmental and other systems will protect you. Will ALL the others in your office or classroom adhere as fully to your strategy as you will? The next circle out would consider people you have to meet from outside your core group. If you have any doubts at all about one of them becoming infectious, maintain your own protective *posture* at a level that will assure your safety.

Cameo-

Two Big Outbreaks in One School

The Middle School and measles outbreaks chanced to begin at the same school (but in different years) Norovirus, probably the cause of the Middle School outbreak, causes gastroenteritis, but is now known to spread efficiently in the air. The most common factor among those who became ill was eating in the cafeteria, even if they carried their own lunch. Spread of measles in that same school seemed almost explosive when compared to other schools. The question was raised as to whether the physical plant characteristics of the cafeteria and its air handling system tended to facilitate spread. That question was not one that could be ethically tested, but the problem became moot when the school was closed, and the building re-purposed and reconstructed.

Reducing your risk in these and other communities may be easier than solving family politics. The same concepts apply. Agreement is best reached by consensus. Those areas where agreement cannot be reached need to be acknowledged, and the implications of the disagreements understood. Where you cannot develop a sense of safety in the community's group behavior, avoid the community, if possible, during an outbreak. If you cannot avoid the community, as may be the case in the workplace, protect yourself as best you can, and try to avoid being the person who helps the disease spread between communities.

It is at the overlap of communities that outbreaks spread and become epidemics if unchecked. By understanding how to break the pattern of transmission at those intersections of communities, you can both protect yourself and help the communities to be safer. If you look back on the way disease spread occurred in the measles Cameo, you can see in hindsight it might have been better to have cancelled sporting events. That would have been considered social distancing. It would have been hard to separate two teenage students in a relationship, and hard to try to stop the spread from one student to a sibling at home, and from there on to another school. Doing so would have entailed either quarantine or isolation of one or more students. In a Pandemic, the resources might not be available to accomplish the detailed epidemiological investigations and interventions needed for control. This is another place where awareness and careful choice of action on your part could help. Self-quarantine and isolation, if needed, can reduce the workload on Public Health staff.

The lesson here is that there can be many factors involved in the spread of infection. There may be places or situations that come to your attention that you will recognize as places you wish to avoid in an outbreak.

Cars, airplanes and elevators are known to be places where person-to-person spread can be facilitated, but certainly these are not the only places to consider. The wisdom of workplace safety rules becomes apparent, and their philosophy may help you focus your thoughts.

Awareness is central to self-protection. Know what is circulating in the community and be aware of any disease control recommendations that have been made.

Know whether any special equipment is needed to prevent exposure. This might only mean having masks and hand sanitizer available for daily activities. You would be less likely to need gloves, eye protection, gowns and booties unless you are directly providing care to persons ill with the disease in question. If you have such a person in your care, particularly in your home, you may need them all. Learn when and where each protective measure should be employed and get in the habit of using them appropriately.

Make sure your house, workspace and other places you spend time do not place you at risk. Do you need to make any changes to your home environment during a community outbreak? For instance, if you have forced air heating or cooling, what kind of filter do you have? Remember that HEPA filter? Is it available so that you can use it to reduce the chance that an ill person coming to your home will infect others? Do you need to increase fresh air ventilation? Are you in a multi-family dwelling where you can separate your air from other dwellings? Do you use an elevator, where the only safe choice is to wear a mask each time you use it? You cannot pay attention only to the places you spend most of your time. Some places, like an elevator at work, may be the highest-risk places you go, even though your time there is minimal.

Cameo-

Leishmaniasis in Iraq

The first year of Operation Iraqi Freedom over 600 soldiers developed "Baghdad boil", or cutaneous Leishmaniasis. Leishmaniasis is a skin parasite that can cause serious organ damage in some forms. It is difficult to cure, so it required special intravenous medication at Walter

Reed Army Medical Center. Conditions were different from what soldiers were used to experiencing. None of the soldiers who became ill knew to worry about sand fleas. As case numbers grew, soldiers began experimenting with their own protective steps, even to the point of putting dog flea collars on their boots. This wasn't effective and was risky for the soldier.

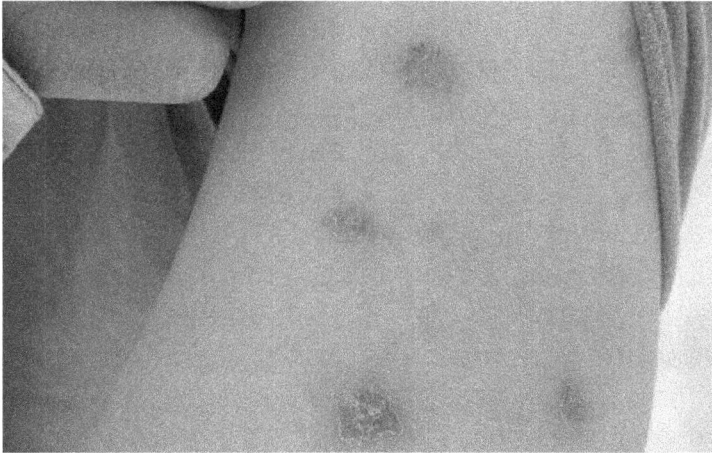

In the first 6 months of the following year, several steps were taken to reduce cases. Treating uniforms with a special insect repellent was a key measure, but "shake and bake", a package of that insecticide a soldier could use to treat his or her uniform, was in short supply. Early in the process, a lecture was given to senior leaders at Balad Air Force Base, home to many units, with the hope that they would take ownership of the issue. Within days, a senior commander came forward and announced that an entire shipping container of the packs had been found in his unit's storage yard. Another senior commander had the newly found packets placed in a self-service supply center where unit representatives collect it easily. The contractor operating the dining facilities put drums of packets at the door to every facility. Units began requesting mass treatment of uniforms for their soldiers by the Preventive Medicine Detachment. Other interventions included identifying and treating areas where sand fleas were present to reduce risk of soldiers being bitten.

The next year, the case load dropped to near zero. Other measures clearly had a role as well, but the overwhelming factor causing the drop was the direct involvement of senior leadership on the base. If the boss pays attention to an issue, everyone else will too.

The message here is that conditions were different from what people were used to experiencing. There were changes that had to be made in the way things were done, and they were made. Both leadership and the people on the ground had to be part of the solution. Government can lay the groundwork, but it is every individual's job to make it work.

Socializing

Socializing can be a significant source of exposures. Whether it is "two ships in the night" meetings with strangers, informal get-togethers for lunch or after school or work, visits to your favorite restaurant or club or events in a closed community, there will be potential for an unwelcome visitor at the party.

Cameo-

The Retirement Community Social

Our jurisdiction had several "over 55" retirement communities of a very high caliber. We were called by one of them when, after a community social event, members started becoming ill. They were afraid that, since the social event was catered, there may have been a problem with the food. The situation was examined carefully.

After the investigation was completed, two things were apparent. First, it was norovirus again, and not the food. By this time appropriate testing was available, and the agent could be determined quickly. Norovirus has a gastrointestinal presentation, so it is not surprising that food was considered first by the retirement community. Next, when the dates of illness were compared, it was apparent that at least one person was ill far enough ahead of the rest to be in consideration as the source of the infection for the rest. Since this person also appeared to have contact with most of the guests, it became even more likely that the outbreak was a rapidly spreading person-to-person outbreak.

The message here is that when an agent is spreading in a community, social distancing can have great value. It also points out the difficulties that can arise when groups meet that have members from other groups. This came from somewhere. Since there was no other cluster in our jurisdiction that could be related to this one, it appeared to be a random occurrence. Since the illness was relatively benign, further investigation was not warranted. If this had been a trade show, and the illness more serious, a much broader outbreak could have resulted from a similar scenario. When you look at your social interactions in your planning, consider not only the possibility of your being exposed at an event, but the implications for spread should that occur. The more severe the disease, the more care you should use in selecting the social interactions in which you choose to participate.

Several cases, to include secondary cases in follow-on cycles, appear to have resulted from one business meeting during the coronavirus outbreak.

What are your plans and *postures* now?

Add any needed components to each of your plans and *postures* to reflect how you would modify your activities outside your home or sanctuary in participating in communities.

Creating safe Enclaves with family, friends, classmates and for work

Your home is your sanctuary or enclave. It is where you feel safe. But we cannot exist as hermits. Work must go on, school must be attended, kids need to play. If you reach the point that the Pandemic is in your locality, and it is causing severe illness and death, you need to be in your most stringent *posture*, adhered to zealously.

Deciding where to venture is difficult. Even more problematic is making that decision for those you are responsible for protecting: Children, the infirm, those needing assistance to go out. Accepting a place as a safe enclave takes trust. If you are dealing with a Pandemic with severe illness and high mortality, it takes life or death trust.

If a Pandemic agent is in your community it is too late to develop that trust. A person afraid for his or her life will say or do almost anything to try to save it. Now, not then, is the time to explore the subject with people you associate with, to get a sense of who you would be willing to join with in sharing safe space.

Family may be the best place to start. If you have multiple generations or branches of your family that you can exchange visits with during a Pandemic, you have a head start. Children may already be going to Grandma's for day care. Grandpa may already be coming to your house when Grandma is out because he wanders otherwise. Two sisters may have a business together operated out of the home of one of them. Siblings may have a long tradition of joint holiday meals. Grandparents may live in Vermont and be willing to take the kids (or all of you) for the duration. Schoolmates may need the continued contact. A school may decide to stay open through the worst of the Pandemic.

If you have a possibility of creating shared enclaves, at least pursue the question. Shared safe enclaves can include any two or more homes where mutual trust allows you to share your homes with everyone that lives in any of them. That is a lot of trust. First, decide what you all want to get out of it. Being up front and honest about it will help you decide if you should pursue the idea.

Next, look at the practical aspects. Can access to the enclaves be controlled enough to protect everyone from an exposure? Can you trust EVERYONE who will participate to not sneak off for a private purpose and become exposed accidentally? Can you physically move from one enclave to another without risk of exposure? Do the physical facilities lend themselves to the purpose? Are supplies available to sustain the population that will use the enclaves? Are PPE and cleaning materials, food and water available?

Assess commitment on the part of all the parties. If everything is still a "go", move ahead with more detailed planning.

Develop a shared safe enclave concept

For each physical space to be used, determine its planned occupancy. Ensure that the physical characteristics of the space will meet the need. Confirm that access can be controlled, and that it can be environmentally isolated from adjoining space. Consider the implications of power loss, failure of a public water supply, or other outside impacts on the viability of the space for this use.

Develop a transportation or movement plan for going from one enclave to another. Becoming exposed on the way defeats the purpose of shared enclaves. Have a plan for what to do if this occurs. How will the exposed person be protected without exposing others in the enclaves? How will you ensure that enclave integrity is not breached? Have rules for when the sharing must end.

Develop common plans and *postures* so that everyone is on the same page at any point. Make sure the plans specify the conditions under which the enclave plans become active. Jointly create a stocking plan for each physical space and decide who will be responsible for obtaining and maintaining the stocks. If a person has special needs materials, they need to be available at every physical space that person uses.

Practice the use of the shared enclave. Rehearse movements and habits. You are all learning how to follow other people's rules and habits while you are in their space. Knowing what to expect ahead of time is important.

Consider whether a self-sequestration space will be created

The highest form of the shared safe enclave might be a self-sequestration space where children, the infirm or others with special needs for protection could live for the duration. The number of people involved, and the size of the space make this very difficult if an institution is not involved. Nursing homes, residential schools and similar institutions come to mind. Such a facility is beyond the scope of this book but might be something you wish to pursue on your own.

Working with Others to Protect Yourself and Your Communities

No man is an island. Society needs to continue during a Pandemic. If you look at your communities as a series of concentric circles as you move out from your family and take in ever larger groups of people, you will find you have a comfort level with trying to work things out with one size of community that you don't have with a larger one. How large or how many communities are inside your comfort zone is a matter for you alone to decide. If you don't have confidence that a community can keep itself, let alone you, safe, then you should try to avoid that community while the Pandemic is placing you at risk. This is easiest to do with social groups, sports teams and the like. Tell them you will be back when it is over.

Housing

What do you find when you step outside the door of your home? If you live in a separate single-family home or a townhouse separated from your neighbor by a firewall, you have a much simpler problem creating your enclave. If you live in a multifamily building with open, outside stairs and hallways, your task is almost as easy. If you live in an apartment, cooperative or condominium structure with enclosed hallways and/or elevators, you have opportunities to work with other residents and the building owner or manager to reduce your risk. The design of the Heating, Ventilation and Air Conditioning (HVAC) system in each building is a major issue.

What do you need to do to prevent your home from becoming contaminated because of the building's design? If you know for certain that your unit does not receive any air from hallways or a shared HVAC system, you can treat your unit as an enclave, and concentrate on safely transiting common space when entering and exiting your unit. This will be the case with many smaller buildings.

I know of one 20 floor condominium where air-conditioned hallways on each floor feed fresh air from the roof to each apartment. Ventilator shafts then carry air from each apartment to the roof. So even though each apartment has its own air handler, any airborne (much more so than droplet) contamination introduced into a hallway by a cough or sneeze could be drawn into any apartment on that floor. One line of defense might be to work with other residents to make the building a shared safe enclave. This would also reduce elevator exposures. Upgrading air filters won't help much here, unless you can filter the air being drawn into your apartment. Blocking the air flow into your apartment has its own hazards and should be considered only after consultation with building maintenance and professional HVAC persons. The best solution will be one adopted for the building as a community. Everyone will have to agree and work together.

Hotels and motels

If you must travel during a Pandemic, find out how your hotel or motel rooms were designed. Totally separate air handlers may be safest, if they have good filters. Shared HVAC as may be found in larger multistory hotels with common corridors and elevators can be a problem. Talk to the hotel before you book. Trying to stay masked throughout your stay is impractical. Your room must be contamination free, regardless of illness being present in other parts of the hotel or motel. If you are a regular, you may be able to work with the hotel manager in advance to achieve this.

Schools

Schools are more difficult. It will be very difficult for a school to guarantee freedom from an infectious student or staff member. As was shown in the community spread of measles, schools were the place of greatest exposure. Be aware of the status of the Pandemic in your locality. Talk to school staff, and work with the Parent-Teacher Organization to find common approaches to protecting students and staff. Many options can be considered.

School systems have plans already. Find out what they are and try to work with the schools. School administrators want to keep school in session, and also keep students and staff safe.

Even if school closure is mandated by higher authorities, you need to keep the educational process in motion. What options for off-site participation do you have? Can the school support homebound instruction? Can you pick up materials for your children? Are courses presented on community TV? Can you work out schedules with other parents to transport children safely if you feel the bus is too risky or is not operating? If too many teachers are ill, do you have skills that can help fill the void?

Children also will need to keep busy during a Pandemic, so that boredom does not turn into unsafe behavior. For some young adult students, helping the community in some way during a Pandemic may be the first real adult thing they do. Can you help organize their opportunity to help this way?

Work

Does your work allow or encourage telecommuting? Is your job one that can be done that way? Can you help your work plan now for continuity of operations if the Pandemic is severe? Many jobs support the infrastructure and must be done by someone. Fire and rescue, police, electricity, water and sewage, trash collection, food provision and heating oil, to name a few, are needed everywhere. If you do not have a high priority job, or are not employed, is there a place you can help?

Do you work for a company with offices in many localities, or for a multinational company? If so, your issues are more complex if you travel for your work or have regular contact with those who do. Much like the airport employee, you must be aware of what may be coming your way from another branch of the company, or what you may find when you travel yourself. A higher level of posture may be needed if an outbreak is underway in a connected location. One consideration would be how long you or another traveler might have to be concerned with becoming ill from a covert exposure. Self-quarantine might be indicated in some instances.

Do you work in a job with high public contact? Workers in convenience stores, for instance, will have a much higher chance of being exposed by an undiagnosed ill traveler than the school secretary. Consider public contact when designing **postures**.

How Government and Response Agencies Work Together in the U.S.

In a Pandemic or other biological event, your first point of contact will probably be by or on behalf of the medical community or Public Health. All jurisdictions have Emergency Response Plans. Most of them cover all hazards and provide for the actions that government will take to assist its citizens in coping with an event. Governments plan to do what is needed, given what they CAN do, for the greatest good of their community. For a biological event, this may not be exactly what each individual needs. In the end, it is you as an individual who must make provision to take care of yourself. If enough individuals do that, the problems the governments must face are smaller.

All responses start locally. If a local government has insufficient resources, it requests assistance from the state. If the situation is beyond the capacity of the state, it requests help from the federal government. The local government and state plans are all under the umbrella of the National Response Framework, which describes how this process is to work, and organizes the way federal resources will be applied. The National Response Framework, which replaced the National Response Plan, provides for the assignment of responsibilities and tasks to federal agencies. It has Emergency Support Functions, such as ESF-8 Public Health and Medical, that provide focus to response functional areas. There is a Biological Incident Annex that outlines the federal response to the types of event discussed here. The Biological Event Annex also describes how bioterrorism events identified by the Federal

195

Bureau of Investigation would be handled, as well as how a response to events first detected by a federal surveillance program would be implemented. All needed responses identified first by the federal government would begin by having a local government response initiated.

The organization charts that accompany these plans show a bewildering array of organizations and agencies. The National Incident Management System (NIMS) is the cornerstone event management methodology mandated by the Department of Homeland Security. Its use ensures every response organization nationwide does things using the same incident management concepts. The plans assign responsibilities and designate tasks, the NIMS effectively links agencies and organizations into a response structure to accomplish them.

Under this system, the Incident Command System is used by local jurisdiction response organizations. In a large-scale biological event, Incident Commands evolve into Unified Commands, and the local, state and federal responses are integrated under NIMS concepts into a national response. This may also happen when any event covers too much geography to be the responsibility of only one state. The response to Hurricane Katrina in 2005 is an example of an implementation of the National Response Plan, the predecessor to the National Response Framework, and the establishment of Unified Commands.

The Federal Emergency Management Agency (FEMA) has a web site where you can educate yourself more fully if you choose. Unless you have a role above local government in a response, your need for detailed knowledge of the National Response Framework and the National Incident Management System is minimal.

Regardless of the scale of the event, your points of contact will principally be local agents. Specialized talent may be called in or requested from a higher level of government. An example might be epidemiologists to track the spread of disease and recommend interventions to stop its spread. With rare exceptions, your locality will remain in control of what is done in the locality. Where in the Hurricane Katrina Response tens of thousands of National Guard went to help, in a Pandemic they will most likely be busy at home. You may really be needed to help your locality.

Many of the responders will be from agencies and organizations with which you are familiar but may be operating in modes unfamiliar to you. If you read your locality's Emergency Operations Plan, at least the portion related to biological events, you can learn of those roles. You will see places you could assist in a response. If you can become involved, do it now so that the ways that emergency response organizations operate will be familiar to you if the need arises.

Non-Governmental Organizations

In a biological event, health care organizations are central to the response. In most cases these will include both for profit and not for profit institutions. Medical Staffs and Medical Societies often have special plans to assist in the community, and of course, private offices will be engaged as well. Many smaller outbreaks are initially identified by private practitioners.

Cameo-

Resistant Strep Throat?

A pediatrician called because of a concern that for the first time Streptococcal throat infections were acting as though they were resistant to penicillin, even when given as an injection to ensure compliance. Strep throat is treated to prevent rheumatic heart fever, a serious illness, so failures to cure could not be allowed.

After calling around, and confirming there was a problem, we conducted a testing program cooperatively with the pediatricians in the community, our Health Department, and the neighboring county's Health Department Laboratory. It was found that a resistant form of Staphylococcus was protecting the Strep until the antibiotic effects ended. This allowed the strep throat to re-emerge. For the next several weeks, all physicians in the community who treated strep throat used a stronger antibiotic. When the Staphylococcus was no longer present, everyone went back to penicillin.

This cooperative effort between the private and public sectors probably prevented a more serious outbreak. Efficiently using this resource is critical.

The Red Cross is one of the most widely respected non-government organizations participating in disaster and emergency response programs. As an organization with national scope, and international sister organizations, it will have a role in any Pandemic. At the local level, it provides many services ranging from shelter management to blood bank services.

Local news media are critical in any response. Getting reliable information into the hands of those affected can save lives in a Pandemic. We were blessed with our local and regional media.

Local Jurisdiction

Local jurisdiction agencies typically include elected and appointed officials in emergency manager roles. Health Departments, rescue squads, police and sheriff, social service and mental health agencies are key players. Public works, information system agencies and school systems may be called into service to provide everything from mapping to transportation to shelter and medical care overflow space. The Fire Chief is almost always the Incident Commander for events in the locality, but in events spanning jurisdictional boundaries, a more complex structure called a Unified Command is instituted. Unlike the Anthrax letters, which defined incident locations, a Pandemic would be geographically dispersed, and a Unified Command used. Larger jurisdictions often have full time emergency response staffs and man full time Emergency Operations Centers. You should know what your jurisdiction has implemented, know how to contact it, and how to get information from it.

States

State law, together with implementing regulations, provides guidance in several areas. For most matters, health is a state issue. Infectious disease, infectious waste and restaurant regulations all help the Health Department reduce risk for the average person. In Virginia, the book "Control of Communicable Disease in Man" (now called the "Control of Communicable Disease Manual") was implemented as law. Other statutes set up the Emergency Response system for the state. There are several authorities for the State Commissioner of Health set down in the law, some of which are delegated to local Health Officers. These authorities provide for quarantine and investigations involving health matters, for example.

States have an important role in biological events. Surveillance for disease and epidemiological investigation are critical during a biological event. Few local jurisdictions can afford to keep the range of skills and numbers of specialists on staff that would be needed to respond to a major event. The state is often the first level of jurisdiction large enough to learn of the number of cases needed to raise suspicion of an outbreak. When an outbreak occurs in a locality, the state, perhaps through regional staff, is the first back up for local staff. The State Laboratory provides a wide range of services often not available locally, and in most states is tied into a national Laboratory Response System with CDC. Virtually all agents that are known to have human epidemic potential can be identified at the state lab.

Each state has its own way of doing business. These ways of doing business are set down in law, regulation, policy and plans. Most of the documents that would cause or allow actions that would affect you during a response to an event are available, many of them on the internet.

National

The Federal Government has many roles in biological events. The Department of Health and Human Services (HHS) is the coordinating agency for biological events. Under the HHS, the National Institutes of Health, the Centers for Disease Control and the Public Health Service fulfill a range of responsibilities going from research to response and enforcement. Surveillance and investigation are accomplished by the Epidemiological Intelligence Service of CDC and by one or more of the Centers. The CDC operate intervention programs for diseases such as Tuberculosis and West Nile Virus. Quarantine at the border and between states is a Public Health Service Function. The Occupational Health and Safety

Administration ensures worker safety in health care institutions and other workplaces. All of these agencies work directly with the states and some larger localities. The list of functions is endless.

In an actual event, the Federal Government operates under the auspices of the National Response Framework described above. It describes how this type of event will be managed, how states are assisted, and how resources will be allocated. It is under this plan that the Strategic National Stockpile is called into play.

Cameo-

The Strategic National Stockpile at Hurricane Katrina

During the response to Hurricane Katrina, over 50,000 National Guard soldiers and airmen were deployed to assist the affected communities. Unlike Public Health Service and Active Military forces, National Guard units only maintain stocks of pharmaceuticals when in Active service.

Many Guard health care providers deployed and set up shop, but were short the supplies they needed to support either the deployed Guard units or the community residents whose own providers and pharmacies had lost their stocks in the hurricane. The SNS deployed, and distributed pharmaceuticals until the situation stabilized. The U.S. Marshall Service provides security to the SNS and was there as well.

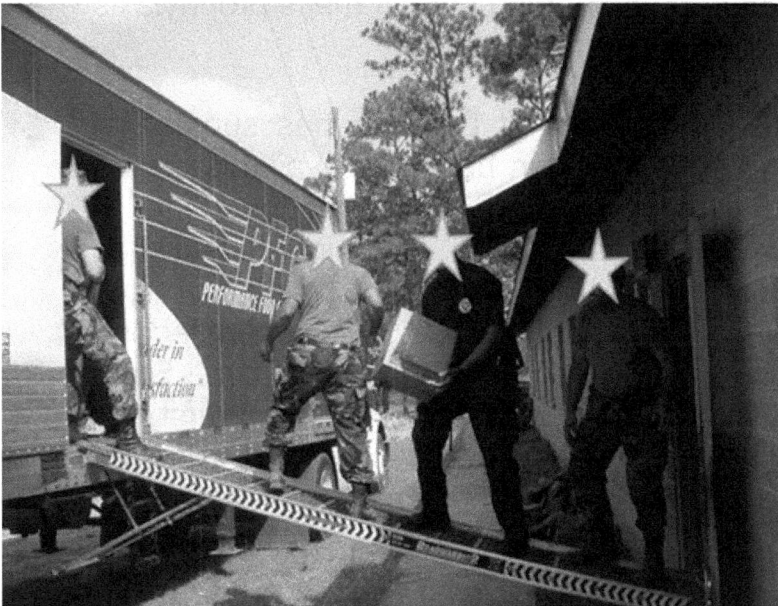

The Strategic National Stockpile is an example of a resource that was implemented with great foresight. When planning for a bioterrorism event made it clear that there would likely be major shortages of medical supplies ranging from bandages and antimicrobials to respirators, supplies were procured and placed around the country so that no area would be long without resupply. The SNS was used to good effect in both the Anthrax event in Washington, and during the Hurricane Katrina response. Plans are now in place for direct delivery of pharmaceuticals to every home needing them if mass prophylaxis ever becomes essential.

The Department of Defense has substantial resources that can be made available during an event. The NRF describes how this is done. Planning for a biological event has considered a range of needs from transportation to medical, and when federal assets are used to augment states. State National Guard assets will be used first, for instance, with DOD resources requested by the state when its own resources are overwhelmed.

International

The World Health Organization is the directing and coordinating authority for health within the United Nations System and is responsible for providing leadership on global health matters. WHO has a vision of an integrated global alert and response system for epidemics and other Public Health emergencies. It acts as a coordinating body.

The U.S. interacts with other nations through diplomatic efforts, through military to military exchanges, and through private enterprise. These channels provide opportunities to facilitate agent spread in a Pandemic, but also channels for support and the flow of information.

What About other Countries and Cultures?

This book has been directed at the needs of the U.S. and takes into account its unique jurisdictional structure. Other countries may have fewer levels of government and provide for emergencies differently. There are four groups that by nature are suited to the major tasks of response, regardless of country or culture. Parts of one task may be accomplished by one group and the rest by another.

Public Health

These functions include surveillance, agent identification, development of control programs and execution of the disease control measures adopted. Enforcement of those measure, to include border control, may be accomplished by the police function. Depending upon the structure of the Public Health and Health Care groups tasks may belong to one group or the other. Functions such as agent identification, for instance, may be accomplished by Health Care.

Health Care

The patient care aspects of outbreak response are provided by this group. Provision of immunizations and prophylactic antimicrobials may be a function of Health Care or of Public Health.

Police

In the broad sense used here, the Police Power includes security and enforcement measures in Pandemic control, as well as more common elements of response. For simplicity, fire suppression and rescue functions are included here, recognizing that rescue functions could just as well be situated with Health Care or Public Health.

Communications

While the news media immediately comes to mind, government must also communicate with the people, and the other three groups with each other. Good quality information must flow in a timely way along several pathways.

If you live elsewhere

Try to take what has been said throughout this book and think of it in terms of how things would have to be done where you live. You may find that what is done by government and other response organizations is much like what you would see in the U.S. On the other hand, it may be so different that gaps will be apparent to you. If you see gaps, consider trying to help close them.

Consider what would need to be done, and who would do it as part of your planning effort.

Working with response organizations

Agencies

Local, regional and state governments all have agencies that do business with the general public on a daily basis. Emergency response plans outline the roles and responsibilities of these agencies in emergencies. Those with roles in a Pandemic will be identified in that section. Look at your local government plan and be aware of your sources of help and guidance in a Pandemic. Know also what these agencies may ask of you. Controlling a Pandemic may involve formal programs of quarantine and isolation, for instance. Rescue Squads may operate under different priorities. Be aware.

Many government organizations rely upon volunteers. Depending upon the size of your community, who you would call to find out who is needed could range from the town manager to a full-time volunteer coordinator. Most volunteers receive training, so becoming involved before a Pandemic occurs would make your help more useful.

Community organizations

The Red Cross is probably the most well-known emergency response non-governmental organization and has a role in virtually every emergency response plan in the country. Almost all their response capability relies upon volunteers. They have training programs for everything that they do. If you have time to volunteer, this is a good place to start.

Many other organizations will be identified in your locality Emergency Response Plan. Health care facilities and medical personnel are key players in a biological event. Restaurant organizations may be providing food to the housebound. If you are in a business that could meet a need during a Pandemic, and your industry is not yet involved in the plan, discuss the possibilities with someone in the Emergency Management function in local government, or with someone in a related agency or organization.

Community activities

One area of need will probably be support of shut-in people who may not have the usual services of their caregivers. Will everyone have food and water, medical supplies, and other needs of living met? While Social Services or a Non-Governmental Organization like the Red Cross may operate programs for this purpose, they will need volunteers. Too many stops for one person creates a risk of more exposures if that person becomes ill. How can you help?

In planning how to meet some of the needs for help that will arise, consider all sources. If the schools are closed, there may be several young adults ready to take on adult responsibility in ensuring the wellbeing of others. If you have young adults in your family, consider whether they could help.

There are many known needs and predicted problems in the Response Plans at all levels from local government to National. Many of these needs could be met and problems could be resolved by people from the grass roots taking ownership for them and working together to get it done. See what roles you could fill in a Pandemic and prepare yourself to fill them. Don't do it alone, do it with your friends and neighbors. Work with the existing agencies and organizations. Be part of the solution.

At a time like this, the good you do will come back ten-fold.

Cameo-

Katrina: Neighbors helping neighbors

When I went to Mississippi and New Orleans as part of the National Guard response, I was amazed at just how much was accomplished by the responders. A unit, mostly composed of soldiers recently returned from duty in Iraq, was sited at a high school in the Southern part of New Orleans. The First Sergeant took me around and showed me what they had done to their temporary residence. They cleaned the school, including the reefer full of rotten food. They repaired the electrical wiring, the air conditioning and the sewage pump. When they were done, the school was operational again. The teachers were gone? Not a problem. They could teach too. Across the street, the Fire House had "Fort Apache" spray painted on its doors. Passers-by had been shooting at the Fire House. The soldiers fixed that. They had been convoy escorts in Iraq and knew what to do with bad guys. After they had arrested a few, the shooting stopped.

Later, I met an officer in the headquarters for the Guard in New Orleans. He said they were having trouble getting the Parishes to release their National Guard Units so they could go home. It seems the first ones to release theirs had the crime rate go back up. The Parishes weren't looking at the Guard units as occupiers. They were friends and neighbors "come to help". There was a cartoon by Kirk Walters that really made that point.

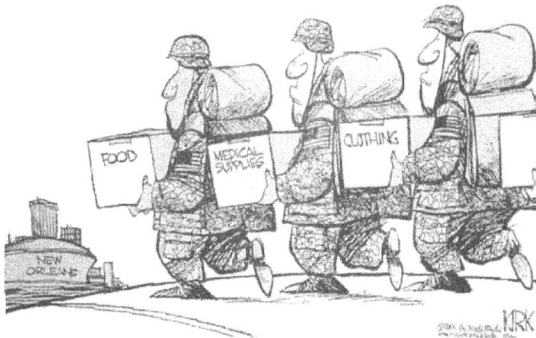

THE SAINTS GO MARCHING IN

FOOD MEDICAL SUPPLIES CLOTHING

NEW ORLEANS

Copyrighted cartoon by Kirk Walters. Used with permission

Working with the news media

The News Media as a source of information

The news media first and foremost is an information distribution community. Its job is to get the word out. It is very willing to print or show information of benefit to the community, and will work with individuals, officials, organizations and locality press offices in finding the best things to propagate. There was a real effort by the media in our jurisdiction to keep things in perspective. At various times we had regular columns in local papers, and a weekly TV show made up of videos on health topics shown on local cable. For a few years, we had local physicians edit California Medical Association Fact Sheets to show the local point of view, and one of our papers printed them in a weekly column crediting both the CMA and the physician.

The support of the media in the Meningitis incident has already been described. When rabies was at its peak in local wildlife, it came through again.

Cameo-

Three Cats

One February, three families were exposed to Rabies by cats. One had been adopted from the local Animal Shelter. Another came from a local Pet Store but had been donated by a local farm to the store. The third was a stray the family had adopted. All three bit a member of their family, were quarantined, became symptomatic, and when tested were found to be rabid. At that time there were many stray cats in the community, often living near dumpsters where they could find food. These tended to be feral cats not amenable to adoption but living in situations where they could expose people to Rabies if they became ill. We instituted a general "cat quarantine" to keep pets in the house. Feral cats were to be trapped and removed from the community. Pets were to have their rabies immunizations brought up to date.

When our plans were announced, the Washington Post chose to treat it like a public service announcement. The other newspapers, and the TV news channels followed suit. The community response was almost unbelievable. Local veterinarians told us that they had immunized about 3000 cats, some they had not seen for 10 years. About 200 feral cats were trapped in the community.

When I went through the line at the grocery store, the cashier asked me "when are you going to let my cat out?". When I went to the Fire Department's annual Steak Dinner

Fundraiser, the Chief came over and jokingly told me his wife said he couldn't feed me until I let her cat out. I went with my daughter to pick up Girl Scout Cookies at a local house. When the owner opened the door, the cat zipped out. His wife called out from the back to catch the cat, but he told her he would watch it. Then he turned to me, not knowing me from Adam, and said "we have a cat quarantine". The objective evidence, such as the large number of immunized cats, and the anecdotal evidence related above, together show the overwhelming impact of the media on the community. Without media support, we could have done little. Because of it, it was a long time before we had another human rabies exposure, and then it was not by a cat.

The news media will work with you if they trust you. Trust is not built overnight. For years, we made it our policy to always respond immediately to the media. It is your best chance to get your viewpoint on an issue out to the public. You may not always like what is reported, but it will almost always be fair. In some cases, they will editorialize in a way that supports you to keep things in balance.

Cameo-

The First Student with Aids

Early in the AIDS epidemic, one of our newspapers decided to print a "For and Against" set of pieces on "Should a teacher with AIDS be allowed to teach". What they did not know was that the School Board was just then considering the enrollment status of its first student with AIDS. Unable to participate by writing the "For" piece for obvious reasons, I was also in a dilemma as to how to handle the fact that the series was going to come out at just the wrong time. In the end, I could only ask the publisher if he could hold off for a week without me giving a reason. The paper agreed. A week later, after the School Board had announced the presence of the student in the school system the newspaper printed its series. It also editorialized in support of the decision of the School Board. The editorial defused any controversy that might have arisen otherwise.

If you have an interest in working with the media, there are opportunities to become involved. During any Pandemic there will be much information to get out, and many questions to be answered.

More and more, the news media are relying upon information feeds from the community, both directly and via social networking. You may be able to be both an information source and an information user through one or both mechanisms. If this is a direction you want to go, contact your local media to find out what options are available.

Media Response to the Outbreak

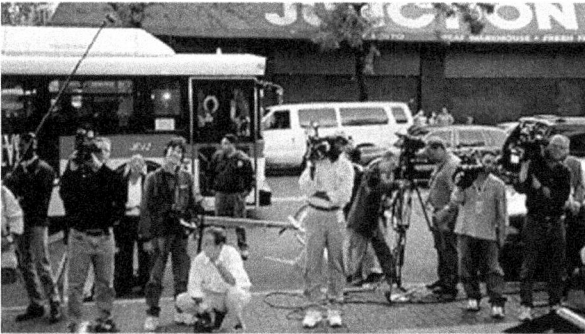

CDC

If you make yourself knowledgeable and develop relationships both with the media and with the response community, you can be a significant force for good.

Where Do You Fit In?

At this point, you should have at least sketched out some plans in your head, thought about some *postures*, and considered how a Pandemic might unfold around you. It is time to consider the how you think of yourself in terms of the roles you see yourself filling.

Yourself

Hopefully, you see yourself first and foremost as a survivor. If you are so unlucky that you become the first person in the world to come down with the new, 100% fatal disease, at least you will get a case report in a medical journal. On the other hand, if you are not that first case **ever**, your chances are much better of never becoming a case at all. By being aware and prepared, you can be proactive in your management of your own safety.

Family

Are you a decision maker in your home? Can you influence the decision maker? Even if the answer to those questions is "no", things might change. Remember what I said about credibility? Other members of your family will either learn about this themselves or turn to you for your expertise if a Pandemic occurs.

If you are the decision maker, think about what a leader does. Some family members cannot be pushed at all but can be led.

Continue to build your credibility in this area, but don't try to force the issue. If you stay aware and advance your plans and *postures* at the right times, things will go well.

Community

Communities need two things. Leaders and followers. There is an old saying that tells you to lead, follow, or get out of the way. You may be a knowledgeable follower in all your communities, or a leader in one or more. Try not to be one of those always in the way. The more credible you are, the more likely your help will be sought out. If there are communities important to you that have a leadership vacuum, fill that void. If you do not have the time, confidence, or skills to do it yourself, use your knowledge to support someone who can.

Business

Businesses will have special needs if they are to remain functional during a Pandemic. Do you have a job that will be essential? Can you help make your workplace safer? As in other communities, leadership is important.

Leadership roles are more well defined in business than in a lot of other communities, and often have the authority to ensure practices that will keep employees safe.

Government

I have met several individuals in government who have been forces for good. It is a worthy goal to be one of them. If you can influence plans and preparations, regardless of your level of government, spend that influence wisely. Hopefully what I have outlined here supports everything you are trying to do. Hopefully, others who have read this book will come forward to help forge the missing links between the public and private sectors, and the everyday people sector. This will both make your job easier and make effective and efficient use of what you provide in a Pandemic.

If you are a first responder, community leader or someone else with responsibility for others

First Responders and other responders

If you are a first responder, thank you for everything you do. When we were putting together the Bioterrorism plans for the Washington, D.C. area, it was the first responders, the police, fire departments and rescue squads who would likely be the first to be in contact with the problem. Not only did they have to do their jobs in a threatening environment, they had to worry about what they might take home to their families. Plans included the best protections that could be devised for the first responders and their families.

The question is debated as to whether first responder families should be at the front of the line for any protections. To me, the answer is clearly YES. Not only are they put at risk by their services to the community, but their families are placed at risk if their protections on the job fail. In addition, they

225

are often volunteers whose families must accommodate their absences at a time they are wanted and needed at home.

In a Pandemic, the risk broadens. Health Department field workers, Emergency Room and hospital staffs, and Shelter staff are among the many groups of people who will be taking on extra risk because of their responsibilities to others. Planning for that situation has extra dimensions.

If you are one of them, planning for your family in your absence is just as important as planning for your own safety. Does your family have its plans and *postures* rehearsed? Can they implement them while you are gone? Have you provided for re-entry in a way that makes them feel safe? Do you have a plan in case you are exposed? Will your role entail a long separation? If there is not a formal plan in your organization around these issues, it may be time to formulate one.

Health Care Workers

The first issue you have to deal with is the need to provide care to people who may be very sick and infectious. The medical community is way ahead of the rest of the country on preparing to deal with infectious disease. If the time comes you have to deal with a real Pandemic, there is a potential for fear becoming a problem for some of your colleagues. Diseases like Ebola can be terrifying, but that terror can be reduced to a healthy fear that makes you cautious but does not reduce your performance. This is a time you can be a role model as well as an educator.

Cameo-

First AIDS patient

When AIDS was new in our community, one of our first cases was someone referred for Home Health services. The nurse assigned to this patient was a professional, well experienced, compassionate nurse. It became apparent that she had misgivings and some fear associated with taking on a patient with this new (to us) disease. Knowing that the patient probably had misgivings as well, I went along on the first visit and took the lead in welcoming the patient to our service. Once I had examined the patient and showed the patient there was no fear or other reluctance on our part to provide the service, and showed by example to the nurse that there was nothing to be feared in laying hands on a patient with AIDS, all misgivings evaporated. We went on to become a significant provider of services to persons with HIV in the community.

An issue that came up during Pandemic Influenza planning was health care system overwhelm. In a Pandemic, there may be simply too many very ill people for the system to accommodate them all. Have you thought about what this will mean to you as you do your job? Is there an organizational plan to deal with this? How will the overload be cared for? Are the answers ones you can live with, let alone be comfortable with? Preparing for this eventuality is not just an organizational issue, it becomes a personal issue when things get bad. Know who will provide emotional support to you should the problem occur.

If you are a health care leader, consider broadly how the resource can be used to best advantage. The overwhelm problem has been considered widely, and several options have been considered in different communities.

Community Leaders

What does your organization expect will happen if people fleeing the Pandemic come to your community? Since some of these people may be exposed and incubating disease, there is risk involved. The impact of an unexpected population to feed, bed and care for must also be considered.

This may be an area where both first responders and non-first responders need to have an expanded role. For instance, can you train and empower rescue squads responding to illness in the home to diagnose, treat, quarantine and isolate in the home as needed? If the Emergency Room and Health Department are both on overload, it could provide medical care and disease control otherwise not available. If it is for your organization, now is the time to reach out to see who will be available in a time of need, and what your true role will be.

Leaders in Business

Businesses that must remain functional during a Pandemic have additional issues to address. You should look at the workplace and see how to make it as safe as possible for employees. The same hierarchical approach OSHA uses for blood borne pathogens can be a help.

1. The more you can accomplish by making sure the air is safe, and workers have enough separation to minimize exposures, the more protection you afford them.

2. Providing PPE and hand sanitizer for use at work, while commuting, and even for at home can keep you in business by protecting your workforce. Helping protect your employee's families will reduce your chance of losing a key employee to illness in the home, or by exposure in the home.

3. Telecommute as many employees as possible. An employee who is safe at home will be less distracted by fear of personal and family risk and may be more productive as a result. Planning for this ahead of time will

incur costs but may result in reduced office space costs over the long term.

4. If some of your employees have a high level of contact with the public, make extra efforts to protect them. Think of the special problems someone like a convenience store worker would have. Besides the OSHA and the humanitarian issues, there is the very practical issue that if you lose your public contact employees, you may be out of business. Look at ways to minimize internal exposures if one of your employees becomes ill.

5. Consider programs to educate employees, and possibly their families, on the Pandemic. The more confident they are that they can protect themselves and their families, the more likely they are to continue working.

6. Maintain a good awareness of the situation and share it with employees. If you can remain calm and thoughtful, you will keep credibility as a good and effective leader.

If you have a business with geographically separated or international branches you have a larger set of problems. In addition to having to ensure the effectiveness of local managers in fulfilling the business leader role described just above, you must consider the impact of travel and transportation on your employees and yourself.

1. Business travel by air may be risky. Consider the frequency and mode of travel and adjust as possible to minimize employee exposures. An employee both away from home and ill will need extra support. An employee returning home ill can expose others upon arrival. Consider minimizing traveler contact with other employees for the length of time recommended as a quarantine period for the Pandemic disease, if an outbreak is in progress and the employee could have been exposed while away or in transit.

2. Businesses with a major function of moving people or goods should look at the potential for facilitating the spread of the Pandemic. The driver of a long-haul truck stops to eat, meets with staff at transfer and delivery points, and otherwise has a potential of spreading illness widely if ill. Make sure each is trained in self-protection and provided with the necessary supplies.

3. A bus, train or airline has a great potential for spreading the Pandemic. Several people will be in a closed transport for some time. One person incubating the illness could expose several other people. Each of these could then further spread the infection as they move to their destinations. You should consider programs to screen passengers before loading and empower employees to deny the obviously ill from transport. Also consider what should be done if a passenger becomes ill during transit. A number of major carriers already do this.

4. Consider the emotional impact one traveling employee becoming ill will have on the rest of your traveling workforce. Consider the impact on home and branch offices, and their willingness to see anyone arrive. An awareness program for all employees on how traveling risk will be managed might go a long way to minimizing employee fear.

Much guidance has already been developed for agencies and businesses by the Centers for Disease Control. Look at the materials available on their website (www.cdc.gov) and consider your operations in the light of what is recommended.

When the Safety Net Falters

If so many are ill that services diminish

Plans usually provide for the possibility that medical needs will overload the medical capacity. Part of what we are must do is prevent an overload by increasing the numbers of people who will protect themselves and not become ill. There are several strategies considered for use if overwhelm does happen:

1. Triage patients. Triage is a sorting process to separate those that will get well from those that will not. Further triage of those who will get well to identify those needing emergency care and those needing care eventually is common. The intent is to use scarce resources to care for as many as possible.

2. Treat at non-hospital facilities. Since hospitals will still have to handle everything from heart attack to appendicitis, creating out-of-hospital temporary wards, perhaps with reduced staffing and equipment is another possibility.

3. Treat at home. This option has much merit when disease severity will allow it, when the risk to those who are at home and still well is minimal, and when needed supplies can be distributed to the homes involved.

4. Adopt reduced standards of care. If the system fails, a lot of people will get no care at all. There has been a lot of discussion about if and how to adopt a standard of care that may not be what we expect now, but which would significantly reduce mortality overall.

Look at your local government plan, and your local hospital plan to see what they have chosen to do. Consider what you would have to do yourself in case the need arises. If needed, rethink your stocking plan. You might be able to care for an ill family member without significantly changing what you have already provided for.

Coping with shortages

Medical care may not be the only shortage. If the Pandemic is severe, loss of employees in infrastructure utilities and businesses may result in shortages of food, loss of power, water and sewage, lack of trash collection and the like. During the Hurricane Katrina response, National Guard units distributed food and water and hauled petroleum products, in addition to many other tasks. You should think through the possibilities and decide if you need to add anything to your stocks that would help you if one of your own set of basic requirements cannot be met by the usual source.

Your circle of protection fails

It will be an emotional blow as well as a physical one if you or a family member in your home becomes ill. If you are reading this, you had the intent to be prepared and to prevent this moment. Now what? The answer is that you continue to do the best you can. If you have been able to prepare thoroughly, you may be able to provide care for the ill person, and conduct the isolation, quarantine and sequestration you need to protect everyone else. If you are the one who is ill and can be cared for by others in your home, all the better. If you live alone or have only people who depended on you in the home, you are more limited in your choices. If part of your planning with family and friends provided for cross-caregiving, you have an option. Otherwise it is time to call for help.

Civil disorder

Movies often portray civil disorder as inevitable. Almost every disaster has its predators. Remember the "Fort Apache" example? State and National plans to support local governments provide for assistance in managing civil disorder. By Federal law, the Active Military is forbidden from exercising police power. The National Guard belongs to the governor and can fill the role of assisting local Sheriff or Police forces. Every police force is likely to have planned for this. If you have the qualifications, this may be another place you could volunteer, but this role would have to be agreed upon by both parties in advance.

Personal Security

The question of personal security is one you must consider. If you have planned and executed your plan well, you will look like a survivor to those around you. It is always possible that someone without your foresight will try to rob you, join your enclave, raid it, or destroy it out of spite or envy. Have your own plan for what to do if this happens.

Afterword

A movie named Contagion was released in 2011. It followed the course of an imaginary worldwide epidemic that spread rapidly and had a high mortality rate. If you can, watch (or re-watch) that movie a few months after you finish this book and consider your own plans and preparations in the light of what is portrayed. You might be surprised at how much your perspective has changed, and how much more prepared you would feel in facing whatever the future brings.

Remember also that a purpose of this book was to help you become more able to deal with the fears that an event could bring without becoming terrorized. For that reason, the worst-case scenario was usually presented, so that you could become comfortable that your plans and **postures** would see you through. There was no intent to make you feel more threatened so that you would over-prepare. Think it through and do what is right for you.

Think of what your role would be in an outbreak: As a survivor, a "case", a parent or child of a case, a teacher or school administrator, a fellow worker, a community leader, a religious leader, as part of the response, or whatever other role you might take. Not everyone is qualified for every role, comfortable with a role, or able to function well in ANY role if one they love is sick. Think about your possible involvement ahead of time and prepare for that role or those roles.
If you are willing and able to take a significant role, become engaged now with your Health Department, town physician, or other agent or agency responsible for outbreak management. Engaging now will make your help more valuable than it would be if you just showed up during an event and offered to help.

Terror is a state of mind we can avoid. The rest is just infectious disease, and the medical community will deal with infectious disease.

References

The World Health Organization has information on international goals and plans:

World Health Organization   www.who.int

U.S Emergency Response is managed by the Department of Homeland Security (DHS). The Federal Emergency Management Agency (FEMA) has its own web under DHS, with public involvement welcomed:

Department of Homeland Security www.dhs.gov

Federal Emergency Management Agency www.fema.gov

All response issues, hotlines and guidance for biological events can be found at the Centers for Disease Control. The CDC have several mailing lists and information packages available:

Centers   for   Disease   Control
www.cdc.gov

An example of State web sites is Virginia's
Emergency Management web site. This
show how you can find your locality
emergency manager:

Virginia Department of Emergency
Management   www.vaemergency.gov

An important resource for those wishing to
monitor world-wide infectious disease events
is a non-profit donation-supported service
called Pro-Med operated by the American
Federation of Scientists:

Pro-med   www.fas.org/promed

Remember that websites come and go. You
may have to search a little.

Appendix

The 10:00 a.m. call from the Middle School Principal was acted upon immediately. The concern was multifactorial: We did not know what organism or agent was involved, or just how severe the case would become. Initial actions included calling the Emergency Rooms and local Doctors offices, dispatching Environmental Health Specialists to evaluate the cafeteria and the building, and establishing a CASE DEFINITION so that cases could be separated from the many other illnesses that would typically affect Middle School students. The good news that came in almost immediately was that all those treating the ill students reported a benign, self-limited illness. A few hours of vomiting, and everything settled down. None of the kids became seriously ill. This gave us time for the rest of the investigation.

It was found early-on that the food storage room had recently been treated for pests, so an environmental agent had to be considered and ruled out as well. All of that took time. A mid-day review gave us both answers and more questions and set the tone for the afternoon's investigation.

The insecticide used in the food storage room turned out to be relatively benign. There was no open food in the room, and even single use products like sugar packets were in larger boxes. A discussion with the State Toxicologist put all remaining concerns at rest, since what few symptoms the agent would cause were dermatologic and not gastrointestinal.

No other environmental concerns surfaced. The inspection of the cafeteria found the usual high standards maintained by schools, with no deficiencies of concern. The building was on public water, and there were no nearby sources of air contamination. The building physical plant was in good condition.

The concern that the illness was foodborne could not be ignored. It was decided that a 200-person case-controlled study would have the statistical power to answer that question. Every Nurse and Environmental Health Specialist that could be gathered quickly was briefed, and then sent to telephones to begin interviewing cases and controls. This was a major undertaking. Each case and each control had to be interviewed. Information was collected on illness onset symptoms and course, foods eaten, place eaten and so forth. Data were recorded and compared with the responses of all the other cases and controls. The Chi-Square test was used to compare ill and non-ill cases and controls for each major food consumed in the cafeteria, to include the pizza. The only factor that approached significance was whether the cafeteria was used as a place to eat. No food item came close.

An epidemiologic curve was constructed for the outbreak. Case finding determined that cases had been identified over a period of days, not just that morning, and in persons not associated with the school as well as students and staff. Outbreaks tend to follow one of three patterns. Point Source is where one food item served one time would have people become ill over time, with the plot of cases resembling a bell curve around the mean incubation period of the organism concerned.

A Propagated Outbreak would show a few cases, then an incubation period later a cluster of cases as each original case infected multiple other people. This one to multiple case expansion would continue until the number of uninfected people diminished and the rate of expansion could not be supported.

A Continuous Source outbreak, such as might be seen with a contaminated well, would tend to show a constant number of cases over time, until the susceptible population had been used up.

In the Middle School outbreak, the epidemiological curve clearly showed a propagated outbreak. Further, the early cases were well before the "big day". The large cluster on the day in question is what attracted the principal's attention. The illness had a very short incubation period, about 19 hours. At that time, direct person to person spread of Norovirus was not as common, and testing was unavailable locally even if it had occurred to us. In today's world, it would be one of the first things considered.

The outbreak has several lessons. One is that the physical environment can shape an outbreak. The dense load of people in the cafeteria, probably combined with the nature of the air handler, enhanced transmission in this school above what was being experienced in the community. Another is that if you establish good communications in a particular community, the data needed to analyze an outbreak is more likely to be collectable in the needed time frame. A third is that there is a lot of "noise" in a situation that may have to be resolved. The "pizza rumor" and the treatment of the food storage room added confusion that had to be eliminated. Items like this are emotion laden and may be constant sources of angst if not addressed authoritatively and quickly. Child safety is a high community priority and a media magnet. In whatever role you become involved, try to be a voice of calm and reason.

www.ingramcontent.com/pod-product-compliance
Lightning Source LLC
Chambersburg PA
CBHW070924210326
41520CB00021B/6793